Contents

Contributors

Shubha Allard
Consultant Haematologist
Royal London Hospital
National Blood Service
London, UK

Trevor Baglin
Consultant Haematologist
Addenbrooke's NHS Trust
Cambridge, UK

John Barbara
Emeritus Microbiology Consultant to the NHSBT
Colindale Centre, London
and
Visiting Professor in Transfusion Microbiology at
the University of West of England
Bristol, UK

Liz Caffrey
Clinical Director – Donors
National Blood Service
Cambridge, UK

Judith Chapman
Manager
Blood Stocks Management Scheme
London, UK

Hannah Cohen
Consultant Haematologist
University College London Hospitals NHS Foundation Trust
London, UK

Marcela Contreras
Chairman of Blood Transfusion International
Professor of Transfusion Medicine
Royal Free and University College Hospitals Medical School
and retired
National Director of Diagnostics
Development and Research
National Blood Service
London, UK

Modupe Elebute
Consultant Haematologist
St George's Hospital
London, UK

Peter Garwood
Managing Director
National Blood Service
Brentwood, UK

Patricia Hewitt
Consultant Specialist in Transfusion Microbiology
National Blood Service
Elstree Gate, UK

Beverley Hunt
Professor of Thrombosis and Haemostasis
King's College
London, UK
and
Departments of Haematology, Pathology and Rheumatology
Guy's and St Thomas' Foundation Trust
London, UK

James Ironside
Professor of Clinical Neuropathology
Western General Hospital
Edinburgh, UK

Sue Knowles
Consultant Haematologist
Epsom and St Helier University Hospitals NHS Trust
Carshalton, UK

Sailesh Kumar
Consultant Obstetrician and Gynaecologist
Queen Charlotte's and Chelsea Hospital
London, UK

Kenneth C. Lowe
Associate Professor and Reader in Biotechnology
School of Biology Sciences
University of Nottingham
Nottingham, UK

Brian McClelland
Scottish National Blood Transfusion Service
Edinburgh, UK

Aleksandar Mijovic
Consultant in Transfusion Medicine
King's College Hospital
London, UK

Mike Murphy
Professor of Blood Transfusion Medicine
Consultant Haematologist
National Blood Service
John Radcliffe Hospital
Oxford, UK

Cristina Navarrete
Head of Histocompatibility and Immunogenetics
National Blood Service
London, UK

Helen V. New
Consultant in Paediatric Haematology and Transfusion Medicine
St Mary's Hospital
London, UK

Derwood Pamphilon
Consultant Haematologist and Honorary Clinical Reader
National Blood Service
Bristol, UK

Fiona Regan
Consultant Haematologist/Transfusion Medicine Specialist
Hammersmith Hospital and National Blood Services
London, UK

Angela Robinson
Retired Medical Director
NHSBT
Watford, UK

Neil Soni
Consultant in Intensive Care
Chelsea and Westminster Hospital
London, UK

Dorothy Stainsby
Consultant in Transfusion Medicine and SHOT National Medical Coordinator
National Blood Service
Newcastle, UK

Simon Stanworth
Consultant Haematologist
National Blood Service
John Radcliffe Hospital
Oxford, UK

Clare Taylor
Consultant Haematologist
Medical Director, SHOT
London, UK

Dafydd Thomas
Consultant in Anaesthesia and Intensive Therapy
Morriston Hospital
Swansea, UK

Tim Walsh
Consultant Anaesthetist and Honorary Professor
Royal Infirmary of Edinburgh
Edinburgh, UK

Jonathan Wallis
Consultant Haematologist
Freeman Hospital
Newcastle, UK

Suzanne Watt
Head of Stem Cells and Immunotherapy
National Blood Service
Oxford, UK

Introduction

In this era of super-specialization, it is difficult to find experts writing clearly about the basics of their specialties, making their subjects accessible to other doctors and healthcare workers. I feel that my collaborators have covered the fundamentals of transfusion medicine in an admirable, easy-to-read, comprehensible way.

This fourth edition of *ABC of Transfusion* has been expanded, with changes to previous chapters and four additional chapters to cover topics which are now established in transfusion medicine, such as haemovigilance, variant CJD, blood stocks management, appropriate use of blood and alternatives to allogeneic transfusion, as well as the increasing involvement of the regulatory environment. The wider breadth of the subject shows that this is not an area devoted exclusively to haematologists, but to all those colleagues collecting, processing and screening blood, prescribing blood components, preparing compatible safe blood for transfusion and administering it.

During my visits abroad in the last ten years, it has been rewarding to learn about the many colleagues worldwide who have encountered transfusion medicine for the first time when reading previous editions of *ABC of Transfusion*. Some of them have become leaders in the field as medical doctors, scientists, medical technologists, nurses, managers and marketers.

Blood transfusion continues to be life-saving in special situations, such as massive surgical haemorrhage, post-partum haemorrhage and severe malarial anaemia in young children. In addition, the safety of the blood supply and transfusion medicine have progressed considerably in the last few years. However, as the message from this book shows, we should only transfuse when the benefits outweigh the risks, yet we are still lacking evidence that blood transfusion works, or that it is the best therapy in a number of the clinical situations in which it is used.

I am grateful to the many colleagues who have contributed to this updated edition of *ABC of Transfusion*; they have patiently awaited its long gestation. I have no doubt that they, as well as the readers, will be satisfied with the outcome.

Professor Dame Marcela Contreras

CHAPTER 1

The Blood Donor: Demographics, Donor Selection and Tests on Donor Blood

Liz Caffrey, Patricia Hewitt and John Barbara

OVERVIEW

- A safe and sufficient blood supply depends upon the recruitment and retention of volunteers who have a low risk of infection with blood-borne viruses and have the committment to make regular blood donations.
- Most blood services world-wide are faced with a challenge in maintaining adequate numbers of safe donors.
- Donor selection is designed to select donors who present a low risk of blood-borne infections and to detect any condition which might make donation hazardous to the volunteer.
- Modern donation screening tests assure a high degree of safety for blood transfusion recipients, but cannot detect all infected donors.
- Increasingly stringent donor selection and donation testing lead to a loss of donors and donations.

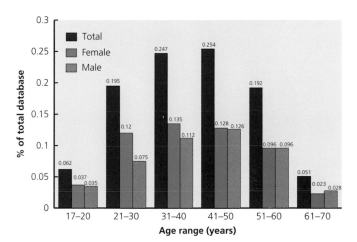

Figure 1.1 Age profile of English donors, January 2005.

Demographics

In the UK all cellular and fresh frozen blood components are sourced from donations made by voluntary unpaid blood donors. A sufficient supply of components for transfusion to patients is therefore reliant upon these altruistic donors continuing to donate. Between 4% and 6% of the eligible adult population donate blood and, in 2005, 1.2 million English donors gave 2.1 million donations. The age range for regular whole blood donation is from 17 to 70 years. New donors are accepted up to their 66th birthday (Figure 1.1).

Donors come from all walks of life but are more commonly from social groups with stable, established lifestyles. Family tradition, peer pressure and personal or professional experience of transfusion are strong motivators.

In recent years it has become more difficult to maintain donor attendance at adequate levels to meet hospital demand. Donor numbers are falling despite heavy investment in recruitment and marketing activity. There are many reasons for this, but the pace of modern living and loss of community spirit are major factors.

Others include lack of time, inadequate opportunities to donate, inconvenient venues and/or opening times, fear of needles and simple apathy. Lack of general awareness of the constant need for blood to support routine medical and surgical treatments is another factor. Volunteers flock to donate at times of 'emergency' but tend not to continue once the perceived need is over.

Donor selection

The possibility that donations might present a risk from transfusion transmissible infections or other conditions is minimized through two essential, complementary steps:

1 Robust donor selection procedures to prevent unsuitable donations from being collected.
2 Routine testing of all donations for markers of infection.

Decisions about donor acceptability and screening tests must take into account the characteristics of the donor population and the prevalence of infections transmissible by blood, the susceptibility of the recipient population, and any emerging risks. Two recent examples of the latter are variant Creutzfeldt–Jakob disease (vCJD) and West Nile virus.

Donor selection has two purposes: to protect the donor from harm and the recipient from any ill effects of transfusion. Potential donors should be provided with sufficient information to allow

ABC of Transfusion, 4th edition, 2009. Edited by Marcela Contreras. © 2009 Blackwell Publishing, ISBN: 978-1-4051-5646-2.

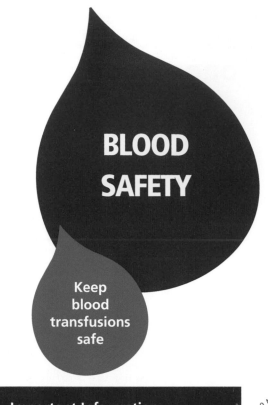
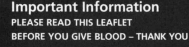

Figure 1.2 National Blood Service blood safety leaflet. (Reproduced by kind permission of the National Blood Service.)

The weight and donation volume limits protect the donor from giving more than 13% of their circulating blood volume, to minimize the risk of vasovagal reactions. The minimum haemoglobin levels ensure that: (i) the recipient receives an adequate amount of haemoglobin (minimum 40 g per unit transfused); and (ii) the donor is not rendered anaemic. Before each donation the haemoglobin level is assessed, usually by a simple, semiquantitative, gravimetric method using a drop of capillary blood introduced into a solution of copper sulphate of known specific gravity. This may be supplemented or replaced by the use of portable haemoglobinometers.

Where the potential donor's medical history or medication indicate that the donor is not in good health or that their own health may be adversely affected as a result of donating, they are deferred either permanently (e.g. in cardiovascular disease) or temporarily (e.g. in pregnancy, anaemia or unexplained symptoms awaiting diagnosis).

Medications are rarely a cause *per se* to prevent donation but may indicate underlying pathology that requires the donor to be deferred.

Adverse effects of donation

Most donors suffer no ill effects. The most commonly reported problem is bruising and/or a painful arm. The overwhelming majority of these donors require only reassurance and simple first aid, unless complicated by infection or nerve injury. Approximately one in 75 donors feels faint during or shortly after donation and 15% of these suffer syncope (rarely serious unless associated with physical injury or slow recovery). These vasovagal symptoms are more common in younger, first time and female donors. Some donors report fatigue in the days following donation. Iron depletion may also occur and blood donation should be considered in the differential diagnosis of unexplained iron deficiency in regular donors.

Recipient safety

The most important consideration in the selection of donors is to avoid the transmission of infectious agents. The voluntary, unpaid status of UK donors contributes to patient safety as there is no financial incentive to conceal relevant details of medical or personal history. In addition, the fact that most UK blood donors are regular donors is an added safety factor.

Donors whose activities are known to be associated with an increased risk of acquiring infections are deferred temporarily for a period that exceeds the incubation period of the infection or, if there is a screening test which is routinely performed, that exceeds the window period for detection by routine screening tests. Deferral is permanent if the activities are ongoing or the infection is chronic, i.e. the volunteer is a carrier of a blood-borne agent. It is very important to exclude individuals whose behaviours are associated with a high risk of acquiring human immunodeficiency virus (HIV), hepatitis B or hepatitis C, and all donors are asked about these sensitive, personal issues each time they donate (Figure 1.4).

In addition, selection criteria take account of other known infectious risks as well as the small (theoretical) risk that may be posed by diseases of unknown aetiology (Box 1.3).

them to exclude themselves; they are required to read essential material before each donation (Figure 1.2).

It is not practical to carry out a full medical examination on every volunteer. Therefore reliance is placed on simple visual assessment and answers to questions about general health, medical history and medication. These are administered using a questionnaire (Figure 1.3) and face-to-face structured interview with a trained member of staff. Confidentiality throughout this process is key to encouraging donors to provide truthful answers. All donors must give informed consent to donation and are required to sign to confirm this before every donation (Box 1.1).

Donor selection criteria

These have been developed and agreed throughout the UK for over 15 years. In November 2005, many selection criteria (particularly with respect to recipient safety) became legal requirements when the EU Blood Directive (2004/33/EC) was incorporated into UK statute (The Blood Safety and Quality Regulations 2005).

Donor safety

Donors must be in good health, within the permitted age range, and meet the minimum requirements for weight, donation volume, haemoglobin and donation frequency (Box 1.2).

Please answer the following questions in blue or black ballpoint pen. If you are uncertain of any answer, leave the box blank and speak in confidence to the healthcare professional.

Donor Health Check for regular donors

A Your lifestyle	Yes	No	Staff
A1 Are you HIV positive or do you think you may be HIV positive?			
A2 Have you ever had hepatitis B or hepatitis C or do you think you may have hepatitis now?			
A3 Have you ever injected or been injected with illegal or non-prescribed drugs, including body building drugs? (You must answer 'Yes' even if it was only once or a long time ago.)			
A4 Have you ever been given money or drugs for sex?			
A5 **To be answered by all donors.** Have you had sex **in the last 12 months** with:			
a anyone who is HIV positive;			
b anyone who has hepatitis B or C;			
c anyone who has **ever** been given money or drugs for sex;			
d anyone who has **ever** injected drugs; or			
e anyone who may **ever** have had sex in parts of the world where AIDS/HIV is very common (this includes most countries in Africa)?			
A6 **To be answered by men only;** Have you ever had oral or anal sex with another man with or without a condom or other form of protection?			
A7 **To be answered by women only;** In the last 12 months have you had sex with a man who has ever had oral or anal sex with another man, with or without a condom or other form of protection?			

B Since your last donation...	Yes	No	Staff
B1 ...have you been told you should not give blood?			
B2 ...have you had an injury which could have put you at risk of hepatitis or HIV (could the virus have entered your body through a needle prick or broken skin)?			
B3 ...have you had acupuncture?			
B4 ... have you had your ears pierced, any piercing to your face or body, had a tattoo or cosmetic treatment that involved piercing your skin?			
B5 ...have you had a serious illness or seen a doctor about your heart?			
B6 ...have you had an operation, any hospital investigations or tests?			
B7 ...have you had jaundice or hepatitis?			
B8 ...has your doctor put you on any medicines, tablets or other treatment (except HRT for the menopause, the pill or other birth control)?			
B9 Have you taken any other medicine or tablets in the last 7 days (this includes medicine you have bought)?			
B10 Have you seen a doctor, dentist or any other healthcare professional in the last 7 days or are you waiting to see one (except routine appointments with your doctor)?			

C Other risks	Yes	No	Staff
C1 Have you had an illness, infection or fever in the last 2 weeks or do you think you have one now?			
C2 Have you been in contact with anyone with an infectious disease in the last 4 weeks?			
C3 Have you had any immunisations, vaccinations or jabs in the last 8 weeks?			
C4 Has anyone in your family had CJD?			
C5 Have you received blood since 1st January 1980?			

D Your travel history	Yes	No	Staff
D1 Have you been outside the UK (including business) in the last 12 months?			
D2a Have you ever had malaria or an unexplained fever which you could have picked up while travelling?			
b If 'yes' have you been outside the UK since then?			
D3a Have you ever lived or stayed outside the UK for a continuous period of 6 months or more?			
b If 'yes' have you been outside the UK since then?			
D4 Since your last donation, have you visited Central America or South America for a continuous period of 4 weeks or more?			

(IN CAPITALS) Forename.. (IN CAPITALS) Surname..
Your Signature.. Date..

Change of details – If we have your details wrong, please give us the correct information below.
Title.................Forename......................................Surname...............................
Address..
Postcode.....................Home no................................Work no.............................
Mobile.....................Email...........................DoB:day........./month........./year.........

Staff Use Only

Other session comments

Accept ☐ Suspend ☐ until........./........./ Withdraw ☐

Medical notes..

Withdraw/suspend until ..../........./
For attention of centre medical staff ☐
Additional letter attached ☐
Set medical bar ☐
Donation instructions...
MO's signature...................Date........./........./

Page 1 of 2 FRM/DSD/CS/004/06

Figure 1.3 National Blood Service donor health check questionnaire, 2006. (Reproduced by kind permission of the National Blood Service.)

Box 1.1 **Donor consent: National Blood Service wording, 2006**

Donor consent should be signed in the presence of a member of National Blood Service staff:

1 I have today read and understood the blood safety and blood donation leaflets. I have been given the opportunity to ask questions and they have been answered.

2 To the best of my knowledge I am not at risk of infection or of transmitting the infections listed in the blood safety leaflet.

3 I agree that my blood donation will be tested for HIV and other conditions listed in the blood donation leaflet. I understand that if my donation gives a positive result for any of these tests I will be informed and asked to attend for further confirmatory tests and advice.

4 I understand the nature of the donation process and the possible risks involved as explained in the blood donation leaflet.

5 I agree to the National Blood Service holding information about me, my health, my attendances and donations, and using it for the purposes explained in the blood donation leaflet.

6 I give my blood to the National Blood Service to be used for the benefit of patients. This may be by direct transfusion to a patient or indirectly as explained in the blood donation leaflet.

Donor signature:
Date:

Box 1.2 **Donor safety: selection requirements**

Weight	more than 50 kg
Age	17th to 70th birthday (regular donor)
	17th to 66th birthday (new donor)
Haemoglobin	>124 g/L (females)
	>134 g/L (males)
Donation frequency	normally 16 weeks (minimum 12 weeks)
Donation volume	405–495 ml (target 470 ml)

Donation testing for markers of infection

Most of the infections that are transmissible by blood transfusion and present a risk to recipients in the UK are characterized by unapparent, chronic or persistent infection. A blood donor therefore presents as healthy, but is capable of passing on infection through the blood. Examples include hepatitis B and C viruses (HBV and HCV, respectively), HIV and human T cell lymphotropic virus (HTLV). These infections are all characterized by the existence of a persistent viraemia, and can be detected by appropriate screening tests.

You must not give blood if:

- You think you need a test for HIV/AIDS or hepatitis.

You must never give blood if:

- You are HIV positive.

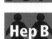
- You are a hepatitis B carrier.

- You are a hepatitis C carrier.

- You are a man who has **ever** had oral or anal sex with another man, even if you used a condom or other protective.

- You have **ever** received money or drugs for sex

- You have **ever** injected, or been injected with, drugs; even a long time ago or only once. This includes body-building drugs. **You may be able to give if a doctor prescribed the drugs. Please ask.**

You must not give blood for at least 12 months after sex (even if you used a condom or other protective) with:

- A partner who is, or you think may be:
  - HIV positive.
  - A hepatitis B carrier.
  - A hepatitis C carrier.

- (If you are a woman) a man who has **ever** had oral or anal sex with another man, even if they used a condom or other protective.

- A partner who has **ever** received money or drugs for sex.

- A partner who has **ever** injected, or been injected with, drugs; even a long time ago or only once. This includes body-building drugs. **You may be able to give if a doctor prescribed the drugs. Please ask.**

- A partner who has, or you think may have been, sexually active in parts of the world where HIV/AIDS is very common. This includes most countries in Africa. **There are exceptions, so please ask.**
Please read the next page

Figure 1.4 UK high risk exclusions as detailed on the National Blood Safety Service blood safety leaflet. (Reproduced by kind permission of the National Blood Service.)

Box 1.3 **Recipient safety: other exclusions**

Permanent
- Chronic infections, e.g. Chagas' disease, brucellosis
- History of malignant disease
- Ulcerative colitis
- Blood transfusion in UK since 1980 (vCJD risk)
- Recipients of human pituitary hormones (CJD risk)
- Recipients of corneal, scleral or dura mater grafts (vCJD risk)

Temporary
- Skin piercing
- Travel to malaria endemic countries
- Surgery
- Flexible endoscopy
- Acute infectious disease
- Immunization with live vaccines
- Dentistry

Currently, UK blood donations are screened for the presence of:
- hepatitis B surface antigen (HBsAg)
- HIV infection, through the use of combined antibody/antigen detection tests with supplementary genomic testing on pools of samples for HIV RNA in some areas
- HCV infection, through the use of tests to detect antibody supplemented by genomic testing for HCV RNA on pools of samples
- HTLV, through testing for antibody on pools of samples
- treponemal infection, through specific antibody detection assays.

All these tests are mandatory, and must be performed on every donation using nationally validated assays, with national 'working standard' samples and full process control.

Additional tests may be indicated for certain donors in particular circumstances. The necessity for these tests is usually decided after considering the epidemiology of the relevant infection and the risk presented from the local blood donor population. For instance, testing for antibodies to hepatitis B core (anti-HBc) is performed on donations in many developed countries, but it is not a routine screening test in the UK. It is used, however, for donors who have a higher risk of recent exposure to HBV infection through, for instance, skin piercing. It is also indicated for donors with a history of past HBV infection. A further example of such additional testing would be for evidence of malaria antibodies, as a marker of past exposure and possible continued infection. The decision whether to test depends upon a careful assessment of the potential donor's travel and residence history. A combination of history taking, postponement of donation until some months after the last possible exposure, and a negative malarial antibody test should ensure that malaria is not transmitted by blood transfusion. A second parasitic infection, Chagas' disease, is treated similarly.

There are other infections that may present a special risk to only a subset of transfusion recipients. An example is cytomegalovirus (CMV) infection, which is a particular hazard for immunosuppressed recipients. Despite routine leucodepletion of all UK blood components, which would be expected to substantially reduce the risk of transmission of cell-associated agents such as CMV, screening of selected blood donations continues to be performed to provide a supply of CMV 'safe' blood components for susceptible recipients. In areas of the world where CMV seroprevalence is very high, such a step would be impractical.

Despite careful blood donor selection and donation screening tests, infection may still be transmitted. Rarely, microbial agents that are not associated with persistent infection, and not therefore included in routine screening tests, can be transmitted by blood transfusion. This is usually because a donor gives blood during the incubation period, and examples have been reported for both hepatitis A and hepatitis E. Transmission of bacterial infection (unapparent donor bacteraemia) has also been reported on rare occasions but most bacterial transmissions are due to (exogenous) skin contaminants. Donation during the incubation period of an infection, i.e. during the 'window period' of infectivity, before reactive screening tests were developed, has also accounted for very small numbers of transmissions of those infections for which blood is now routinely screened, e.g. HIV.

Finally, there are infections for which there are no suitable screening tests; for the UK, vCJD is the most significant example. As virtually the whole of the UK population has been at risk of vCJD infection through diet in the past, the development of suitable blood tests and/or prion removal filters is proceeding (see Chapter 14). Thus, although blood transfusions in the UK are exceedingly safe, there still remains a very small risk of transmission of infection, and this fact reinforces the need for testing to be combined with careful donor selection.

Serological testing

Serological tests are carried out on all donations to ascertain the blood group (A, B, AB or O) and for RhD typing; the results are checked against those previously obtained from that donor or by repeat typing with different batches of antibodies and test cells. Most UK centres also test for RhC, c, e, E and K antigens, and this information appears on the blood pack label. Blood units found negative for D antigen are labelled 'RhD negative'. With the monoclonal typing antibodies in current use, most weak and variant forms of D antigen are detected on direct testing. Those below the limit of detection with monoclonal anti-D are labelled as RhD negative since they are not considered to be immunogenic to a D-negative recipient. Extended testing to detect, for example, weak D or D^u in donors is not universally carried out. A proportion of the units is also typed for C^w, Fy^a, Fy^b, M, S, s, Jk^a and Jk^b, thus making the phenotyped red cell stocks readily available for alloimmunized patients in need of transfusion.

All donations are screened for clinically important red cell antibodies. Any donation found to have a high antibody titre should not be used for transfusion, although it may be a valuable source of red cell typing reagent. Low titres of antibodies should not automatically exclude a donation from therapeutic use as the antibody would be further diluted on direct transfusion. As well as this, about 90% of the plasma (and hence antibodies therein) from most donations is removed and the cells are resuspended in an additive solution such as saline adenine glucose mannitol (SAG-M); most of the remaining red cells just have most of the plasma removed (see Chapter 4). The comparatively unrefined antibody screening, possible on automated blood grouping machines, is therefore acceptable in the testing of blood donations, although it is not acceptable in the screening for antibodies of samples from potential recipients. An exception to this is the selection of blood for 'massive' transfusion of a neonate, when donor blood should be screened for antibodies using sensitive techniques.

Testing of group O blood for high titre haemolytic anti-A, anti-B and anti-AB is still carried out in some centres in the UK, so that plasma-rich components, such as platelet preparations, can be appropriately labelled. This practice should not be allowed to override the principle that a patient should receive blood of his/her own group and that group O donor blood (especially plasma-rich components) should not be given to patients of other groups except in an emergency.

In England, typing for human leucocyte antigen (HLA) or histocompatibility antigens is carried out on regular plateletpheresis donors, to satisfy the demand for HLA-matched platelets. Such platelets are used in the treatment of a severely thrombocytopenic patient who, because of many exposures to blood components, has developed multispecific antibodies to HLA antigens and has become refractory to random platelet transfusions. Normally, HLA-compatible donors would provide one or two adult doses of platelets by means of plateletpheresis. Typing for human platelet antigens HPA-1a and HPA-5b is also performed on regular plateletpheresis donors to supply compatible platelets for the transfusion of fetuses and infants affected by neonatal alloimmune thrombocytopenia. Occasionally, HPA-typed platelets are required for the transfusion of immunologically refractory patients with anti-HPA.

Further reading

Barbara JAJ, Regan F, Contreras M. *Transfusion Microbiology.* Cambridge University Press, 2008.

Klein HG, Anstee DJ, *Blood Transfusion in Clinical Medicine,* 11th edn. Blackwell Publishing Ltd, 2005.

Murphy MF, Pamphilon DH (Eds). *Practical Transfusion Medicine.* Blackwell Publishing Ltd, 2001.

CHAPTER 2

Supply and Demand for Blood and Blood Components and Stock Management

Judith Chapman, Peter Garwood and Sue Knowles

OVERVIEW

- This chapter covers the different elements of the blood supply chain.
- Blood supply and component preparation are examined.
- Influences on the demand for blood and blood components are discussed.
- Factors affecting blood inventory management practice are outlined.
- Finally, future influences on the blood supply chain are looked at.

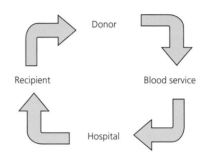

Figure 2.1 The blood supply chain.

Ability to meet the demand for blood and blood components is a primary goal of blood services, and is achievable through the good will of voluntary donors, effective inventory management and the appropriate use of blood and its alternatives by clinicians. The blood supply chain (Figure 2.1) includes the voluntary blood donor, the blood services, the hospital laboratory, the prescribing clinician and the recipient of blood. It is the responsibility of the blood services to minimize production loss and wastage and to employ good inventory management practice in conjunction with the hospital laboratories, whilst clinicians are responsible for prescribing blood only when there are no alternative approaches and the benefits exceed the risks. Blood is a freely given resource and a collaborative approach along the chain is required to ensure that it is available and used for the maximum benefit to patient care.

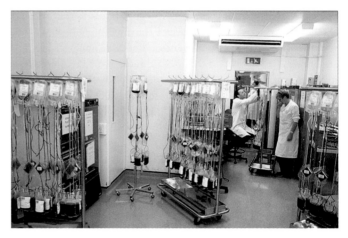

Figure 2.2 The leucocyte depletion process showing red cells undergoing filtration for leucocyte depletion.

The blood supply

Volunteer donors are the source of the blood supply chain; however, the donor base continues to fall despite recruitment efforts. Research in England and North Wales indicates that the active donor base is shrinking. Although the risk from transfusion-transmitted infections has never been lower, the demand for safety through additional screening tests has never been greater. All additional testing for pathogens has the potential to lead to false positive reactions, and further donor deferrals and disqualifications.

The appreciation that variant Creutzfeldt–Jakob disease (vCJD) is likely to be transmitted through the blood supply has led to the exclusion of donors who have themselves been transfused and who are therefore particularly motivated to donate. Increased foreign travel and its associated risks of disease (e.g. malaria and West Nile virus) have also had an impact on the blood supply.

Whole blood donations (450 ml ± 10% of blood) are processed and converted into concentrated red cells and, according to requirements, platelet concentrates, fresh frozen plasma and cryoprecipitate.

In many developed countries, blood undergoes universal leuco-depletion (Figure 2.2) for a number of reasons: to reduce the risk

ABC of Transfusion, 4th edition, 2009. Edited by Marcela Contreras. © 2009 Blackwell Publishing, ISBN: 978-1-4051-5646-2.

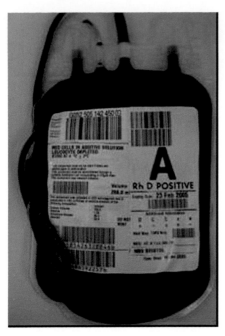

Figure 2.3 Leucocyte-depleted red cells in additive solution.

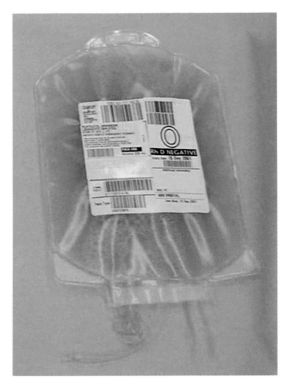

Figure 2.4 Leucocyte-depleted pooled platelets.

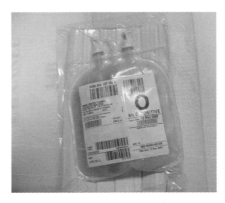

Figure 2.5 Fresh frozen plasma pack.

of transmission of vCJD, to remove leucocyte-associated viruses (e.g. cytomegalovirus or CMV), and to reduce other complications of transfusions related to the white cell content (e.g. the development of antibodies against human leucocyte antigen (HLA)) causing refractoriness to platelet transfusions or problems with future transplants. Following leucodepletion, concentrated red cells are resuspended in an additive solution to maintain red cell viability, to a final volume of 220–340 ml (Figure 2.3). In the UK, concentrated red cells may be stored for up to 35 days, at a controlled temperature range of 2–6°C. Changes that occur during storage include loss of viability, changes in metabolism, a reduction in pH, and an increase in potassium levels in the plasma.

Platelets can either be derived from whole blood donations or by pooling buffy coats from four whole blood donations or from single donor apheresis. In England and North Wales approximately 50% of preparations are prepared by apheresis and 50% from buffy coat pooling. Apheresis platelets are provided for recipients up to the age of 16 years, to reduce the risk of transfusion-transmitted infections by reducing donor exposure. An additional benefit of collecting apheresis platelets is that donors typed for HLA and human platelet antigens (HPAs) can be used to meet the requirements of patients with immunological refractoriness to random platelets and to cater for the specific requirements of intrauterine or neonatal transfusions in fetuses and infants suffering from alloimmune thrombocytopenia. Apheresis platelets undergo the same stringent testing procedures as whole blood donations.

Platelet concentrates (Figure 2.4) are stored in plasma (or platelet storage medium) at 20–24°C, normally for up to 5 days, and must be kept agitated. Platelets have a short lifespan due to loss of viability during storage and the potential for bacterial contamination. Consequently they have their own inventory management requirements. To ensure sufficiency over busy public holiday periods, additional supplies are required. However, with the potential for screening platelets for bacterial contamination prior to issue and the improved storage of leucodepleted platelets, the shelf life can be extended to 7 days to cover holiday periods.

Fresh frozen plasma (FFP; Figure 2.5) is sourced from both this country and the USA. The use of imported plasma reduces the risk of transfusion-transmitted vCJD and is transfused to recipients up to 16 years old. Imported plasma is also used exclusively for the manufacture of plasma products. Because the risk of viral-transmitted infections is lower in the UK donor population than in most other countries, imported FFP needs to undergo viral inactivation. FFP may also be virus inactivated, using either methylene blue (MB) or solvent detergent (SD) treatment. MB treatment can be applied to single packs, whereas SD treatment can only be applied to large pools of plasma. Both methods offer good virus protection but are associated with loss of coagulation factors. MB-treated virus-inactivated plasma imported from the USA is currently recommended

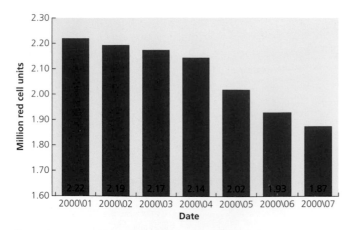

Figure 2.6 Demand for red cells in England and North Wales, 2000–2007.

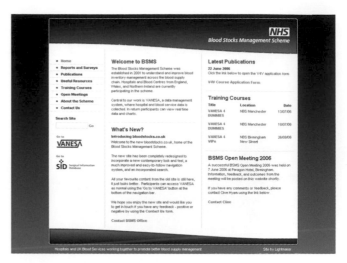

Figure 2.7 Blood Stocks Management Scheme website home page, www. bloodstocks.co.uk.

for recipients up to the age of 16 years, while SD-treated plasma is reserved for patients with thrombotic thrombocytopenic purpura undergoing daily large volume plasma exchange.

Demand for blood components

Demand is difficult to forecast for many reasons, since it follows the net effect of changes in population demographics and the degree of uptake of blood conservation strategies. Tools such as environmental scanning, mathematical modelling and trending can be used to try to forecast demand more accurately. The red cell demand forecast is used to calculate and set blood collection targets, which then form the basis for collection session planning.

There has been a decline in red cell demand in England over recent years and, despite an estimated blood donation rate of about 39 units per 1000 of the eligible donor population (the range for high Human Development Index (HDI) countries is 10.4–74.0), England and North Wales are self-sufficient in red cells. All requests for red cells from hospitals have been fully met by the National Blood Service over the last 6 years. In England and North Wales the demand for red cells has fallen year on year since 2000. In 2000/01 red cell demand was 2.22 million, but in 2006/07 had fallen to 1.87 million, a fall of 15.8% in 6 years (Figure 2.6). Lower demand may be attributable to a number of reasons including the publication of the Health Service Circular (HSC) 2002/09 *Better Blood Transfusion II* (see Chapter 18), the year on year increase in red cell prices, concerns over possible blood shortages, and the establishment of the Blood Stocks Management Scheme (BSMS) (Figure 2.7).

The use of blood during surgery has fallen significantly due to several factors, including improved surgical and anaesthetic techniques, treatment of correctable anaemias at pre-assessment clinics, the use of antifibrinolytic agents, intra- and postoperative cell salvage, and protocols for transfusion thresholds (see Chapter 16). However, successive audits still show considerable variability in the blood used for a given surgical procedure between different hospitals. An increasing proportion of red cells is transfused to medical and haemato-oncology patients, some of whom may be entirely transfusion-dependent. Erythropoietin may alleviate the anaemia

in some categories of patients (e.g. lymphoproliferative disorders or following chemotherapy for solid tumours), but in the absence of recommendations from the National Institute for Health and Clinical Excellence few trusts have opted to fund it. Nevertheless, erythropoietin may reduce the demand for blood in some medical patients with chronic anaemia.

Inventory management

Different factors influence inventory levels in hospitals and blood services. Blood services need to balance the need to have sufficient stock to meet demand against having an excess of stock that leads to older red cells being issued and wastage due to time expiry. High red cell stock levels in the blood services leads to hospitals receiving blood that has a reduced shelf life, giving the hospital less time for the unit to circulate through the reserved/unreserved, stock/issue loop, thus increasing time expiry losses. The National Blood Service in England and North Wales has a policy of moving stock from centre to centre to ensure an equitable supply throughout the country. However, because of the lack of cold chain validation for the whole supply chain including the hospital, stock cannot currently be moved back from the hospital to the blood centre.

Hospitals also need to balance their inventory levels in order to have sufficient red cells to meet clinical demand but not an excess that leads to increased time expiry wastage. Several factors influence a hospital's red cell inventory levels, including its size, the time taken for blood to arrive from the local blood centre, and the presence of specialist clinical units including trauma and orthopaedics.

Laboratory policies may also have an impact on the inventory. The BSMS has noted that, for group O RhD-positive red cells, an increasing reservation period following crossmatching is associated with a higher inventory level and has demonstrated a significant difference between a 24-hour reservation period and longer reservation periods of 48 or 72 hours. It has also shown that hospitals that have replaced the serological crossmatch between donor and recipient with electronic issue have lower red cell issues from the National Blood Service. Electronic issue relies on an electronic check for blood group matching between the red cell unit and the recipient; the security is dependent on the validity of each of these blood groups. The recipient must have been grouped twice with identical findings and have a negative red cell antibody screen.

Hospitals using electronic issue are able to reduce their red cell inventory because less red cell units are tied up in crossmatch fridges and, therefore, stock available for issue can be used more efficiently. Effective hospital inventory management practice includes a 24-hour crossmatch reservation period, use of electronic issue, appropriate stock holding of group O RhD-negative and groups A and AB red cell units, and stock management training.

In addition to time expiry wastage, losses may occur throughout the supply chain for a number of reasons. Incomplete donations may occur because of poor veins, and processing losses include faulty seals and repeat reactive microbiology screening tests (e.g. anti-human immunodeficiency virus, anti-hepatitis C virus). Units may also be lost to the supply chain because they are sent for quality monitoring. Reasons for hospital losses include the unit being left out of a temperature-controlled environment for more than 30 minutes, if the unit is being returned to stock, or a breakdown of the storage fridge.

The future

The future of the blood supply remains dependent upon the altruistic blood donor; the possibility of a flu pandemic or the introduction of a test for vCJD may have a significant detrimental impact upon its availability. Blood services and hospitals have prepared emergency blood management plans in order to try to ensure supply continuity for those patients whose dependence upon blood transfusion cannot be avoided.

The increased use of erythropoietin could help bridge the gap in the event of a supply shortage for some patients. Effective red cell substitutes may provide another solution, but although these have been discussed over a number of years and some progress has been made, much work still needs to be carried out before those in development are brought into clinical use (see Chapter 17).

There is undoubtedly still much to be achieved in educating prescribers of blood to avoid unnecessary transfusions and to consider alternative strategies. Peer review of transfusion practice through national and regional audits of blood component usage and the benchmarking of blood use in common surgical procedures are ongoing, and are to be encouraged.

Further reading

Chapman JF, Cook R. The Blood Stocks Management Scheme, a partnership venture between the National Blood Service of England and North Wales and participating hospitals for maximising blood supply chain management. *Vox Sang* 2005; **83**: 239–46.

Prastacos GP. Blood inventory management: an overview of theory and practice. *Management Science* 1984; **30**: 777–800.

Thomas D, Thompson J, Ridler B. *A Manual for Blood Conservation*. tfm Publishing, Shrewsbury, 2005.

Wallace EL. Monitoring the nation's blood supply. *Transfusion* 2003; **43**: 299–301.

www.bloodstocks.co.uk. For articles on blood inventory management.

CHAPTER 3

Compatiblity Testing Before Transfusion; Blood Ordering and Administration

Marcela Contreras and Aleksandar Mijovic

OVERVIEW

- If tests are done to ensure that the donor and recipient belong to the same ABO and RhD groups, then – even if no other tests are done – the donor's red cells will be compatible with the recipient's plasma in more than 98% of cases.

- Sampling and labelling errors can be avoided by scrupulous attention to patient identification and proper sampling procedure.

- A negative antibody screen and confirmed ABO and Rh groups permit 'electronic' blood issue, reducing the time required for the provision of blood as well as the blood bank workload. A serological crossmatch must be performed for patients with red cell alloantibodies and those who have had organ transplantation.

- A final transfusion check matches the details on the blood bags with those on the blood prescription chart and on the patient's wristband. Electronic identification systems further reduce the risk of transfusing the wrong blood.

- Blood usage in surgery is declining, despite increasingly complex procedures, due to lower transfusion triggers, wider use of blood conservation methods, and advances in surgical techniques.

- A regular audit of blood ordering and usage is paramount in maintaining good transfusion practice.

Compatibility testing (crossmatching) using the recipient's plasma/serum and the donor's red cells has been the standard blood bank approach in preventing the serious haemolytic transfusion reactions that might ensue if the recipient has antibodies directed against antigens present on the donor's cells. Clinical experience accumulated over years, the need to meet an increasing demand for blood in busy hospitals, as well as the impact of pre-transfusion testing on the workload in the blood bank, have led to a review of techniques used for compatibility testing. At the same time, it is mandatory that high safety standards are maintained.

ABC of Transfusion, 4th edition, 2009. Edited by Marcela Contreras. © 2009 Blackwell Publishing, ISBN: 978-1-4051-5646-2.

Ordering blood components and compatibility tests

When the decision is made that a patient needs (or is likely to need) a transfusion, blood samples (anticoagulated with ethylene diaminetetra-acetic acid (EDTA)) should be sent to the blood bank or hospital transfusion laboratory (HTL). The sample must be accompanied by a request form, filled in either by hand or on the computer linked to a printer in the blood bank. Emergency requests can be made by phone: HTL staff must write down all the necessary details on the form specially designed for this purpose.

The request form must contain the name and contact number of the clinician responsible for the patient, and patient identifying details – full name, date of birth and unique hospital number (Figure 3.1). Clinical details should be included, such as the diagnosis, or the surgical operation the patient is scheduled for, as well as the history of previous transfusions or pregnancies. The number of units of blood requested (if any) and the urgency of transfusion, as well as the reason for transfusion, should be stated. The HTL should not accept incomplete request forms. The percentage of samples refused because of incomplete patient details is usually around 5–10%; ordering through electronic patient records is expected to reduce the number of these errors.

Most deaths associated with blood transfusion are the result of mistakes in identification. Some of the mistakes occur at the stage of taking a blood sample from the potential recipient. In an international survey, approximately one in 2000 samples contained blood from the wrong patient. Measures to avoid these errors are listed in Table 3.1.

Blood grouping and antibody screening

Blood grouping

The patient's red cells are grouped for ABO and RhD and the plasma is tested for anti-A and anti-B to confirm the patient's group ('reverse grouping'). This is essential because of the presence of haemolytic antibodies in the plasma of subjects who lack the corresponding ABO antigens. These antibodies can cause intravascular haemolytic transfusion reactions, and even death, in the case of major incompatibility between the donor and the recipient (e.g. recipient group O and the donor red cells group A, B or AB) (Tables 3.2 and 3.3).

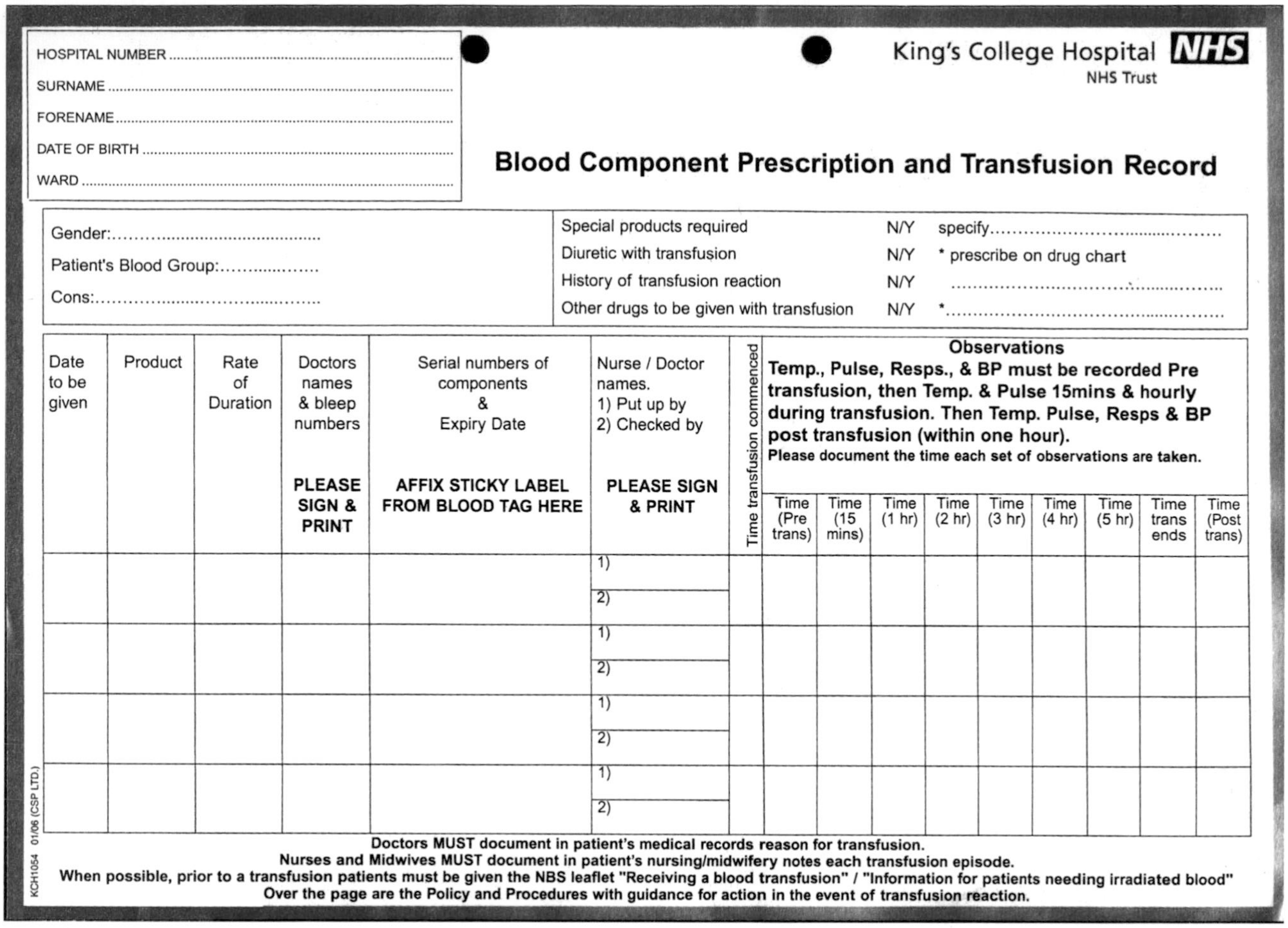

HOSPITAL NUMBER ....
SURNAME ....
FORENAME ....
DATE OF BIRTH ....
WARD ....

King's College Hospital NHS
NHS Trust

Blood Component Prescription and Transfusion Record

Gender:........
Patient's Blood Group:........
Cons:........

Special products required	N/Y	specify........
Diuretic with transfusion	N/Y	* prescribe on drug chart
History of transfusion reaction	N/Y	....
Other drugs to be given with transfusion	N/Y	*........

Date to be given	Product	Rate of Duration	Doctors names & bleep numbers PLEASE SIGN & PRINT	Serial numbers of components & Expiry Date AFFIX STICKY LABEL FROM BLOOD TAG HERE	Nurse / Doctor names. 1) Put up by 2) Checked by PLEASE SIGN & PRINT	Time transfusion commenced	Observations: Temp., Pulse, Resps., & BP must be recorded Pre transfusion, then Temp. & Pulse 15mins & hourly during transfusion. Then Temp. Pulse, Resps & BP post transfusion (within one hour). Please document the time each set of observations are taken. Time (Pre trans)	Time (15 mins)	Time (1 hr)	Time (2 hr)	Time (3 hr)	Time (4 hr)	Time (5 hr)	Time trans ends	Time (Post trans)
					1) 2)										
					1) 2)										
					1) 2)										
					1) 2)										

KCH1054 01/06 (CSP LTD.)

Doctors MUST document in patient's medical records reason for transfusion.
Nurses and Midwives MUST document in patient's nursing/midwifery notes each transfusion episode.
When possible, prior to a transfusion patients must be given the NBS leaflet "Receiving a blood transfusion" / "Information for patients needing irradiated blood"
Over the page are the Policy and Procedures with guidance for action in the event of transfusion reaction.

(a)

Figure 3.1a An example of the blood prescription chart. In addition to patient information and special requirements, it contains data on the blood component requested, and provides a column to affix the label from the blood component, tracing it to the patient. Matching is checked by two authorized persons who sign the chart. The next columns are for recording observations during transfusion.

The RhD antigen is highly immunogenic; once anti-D is formed, it may destroy RhD-positive cells and may also cause severe haemolytic disease of the fetus/newborn. Thus it is important to type women of childbearing age, as well as girls, for RhD before transfusion. RhD-negative subjects are, as a rule, transfused with RhD-negative red cells, but if there is a shortage of such blood, unimmunized RhD-negative men and unimmunized women above the age of 60 may safely be given RhD-positive red cells.

Ideally, girls and women of childbearing age who are candidates for red cell transfusion should also be typed for the RhD and K antigens so that, if negative, they are given antigen-negative red cells, thus avoiding immunization and the risk of haemolytic disease in their offspring.

Some categories of transfusion-dependent patients, such as those with sickle cell anaemia, need to be fully phenotyped before starting transfusions, in order to anticipate potential alloantibody formation. They should be given red cells matched for the most immunogenic antigens, i.e. all Rh (CcDEe) and K antigens.

Antibody screening

To detect clinically important red cell alloantibodies – those reacting at 37°C and capable of destroying red cells that carry the relevant antigen (e.g. Rh, Kell, Duffy or Kidd antibodies) – testing against two or three selected screening cells should be carried out on all patients' plasma/serum samples. The screening cells are always group O and carry, between them, most of the antigens that stimulate the formation of clinically significant antibodies (e.g. D, C, c, E, e, K, Fy^a, etc.) (Figure 3.2). When an atypical antibody (against antigens other than A or B) is detected, its specificity must be defined by testing the patient's plasma against a collection of fully typed red cells ('identification panel'). Testing for red cell antibodies should be done by the indirect antiglobulin test (IAT or indirect Coombs' test), performed at 37°C.

Whenever possible, grouping and screening should be performed well in advance of transfusion, in order to allow time for additional tests and ordering cells of rare blood groups. If the patient has alloantibodies directed against a common antigen (e.g. anti-U), it may take a few days to find compatible blood. In certain cases the national and international bank of frozen rare cells may be the only source of compatible cells.

If patients have received transfusions or been pregnant within 3 months samples should be taken within 48–72 hours; and if patients have received transfusions less than 10 days previously, samples should be taken within 24 hours of the planned transfusion.

COLLECTION	CHECKING 'No ID BAND No BLOOD'	OBSERVATION	REACTION
Only staff who have been trained in the process of collection can collect blood components. Always take prescription or compatibility form to check unit at collection point in Blood Bank. Print your name, date & time on collection form. **Red Blood Cells** Complete infusion within 5hrs. Do not refrigerate if out of the fridge for more than 30mins + transfusion not imminent. **Platelets** Infuse within 30 minutes. Use platelet giving set from blood bank. **FFP & CRYO** Infuse within 4hrs. **HAS** Infuse within 3 hours.	Ensure patient is aware of & given the transfusion information leaflet. When able, obtain verbal consent. 2 professionals to perform **bedside** check Check ID band for Pts full name, unit no. DOB & sex. **Positive Patient Identification** Ask patient their name & DOB **Unit check & Tags** Group, expiry, serial number, time component removed from fridge. Peel off label from Tag and place on prescription chart. Fill out Tag and place in ward box. **Documentation Check:** • Patient ID band • Prescription chart • Compatibility form • Tag on unit • Serial number & Group on unit • Notes **Also check** special requirements. e.g. irradiated , CMV negative. **Flying Squad blood** is O neg & un-X-matched. Blood Bank must be notified immediately of its use & fate	**Record baseline** observations T, P, R & B/P prior to transfusion. **Repeat T & P** at 15 minutes. Most transfusion reactions will occur with infusion of 10-30mls. **Continue hourly T & P** with patient under supervision until transfusion is completed. **Post transfusion (within an hour)** repeat T, P, R & B/P. **Indication of transfusion reaction** Fever Rigor Anxiety Flushing Loin pain ⇓B/P Chest pain Shortness of breath. **Advise patients** to inform staff if they are experiencing any of the above signs and or symptoms. **Guidelines Available** (Kingsweb -Cliniweb –Guidelines-Haematology-Blood Transfusion Services) Blood transfusion policy. Use of Blood components. Elective surgical blood order schedule (ESBOS). Neonatal guidelines. **Document** rationale for transfusion and products transfused in medical records & nursing/midwifery notes.	If a transfusion reaction is suspected, **STOP** the transfusion. Recheck the pts. identification and compatibility of the unit. **Mild reaction:** E.g. Temp rise less than 1.5°C +/- urticaria but nil else. Liase with doctor for symptom control with anti-pyretic & antihistamine. Transfusion may continue but increase regularity of observation. **Severe reaction:** E.g. Temp rise more than 1.5∞C or patient is otherwise unwell. Discontinue the transfusion and notify the doctor. Treat symptoms. Observe patient for shock. Treat as appropriate. **Do not transfuse any further blood products.** **Initial follow-up to severe reaction.** • Notify Blood Bank ASAP. • Return suspect unit. • Refer to Haematologist. • Repeat Group and Xmatch. • Send 2 EDTA & 1 Clotted samples for DAT (direct antibody test). • Blood Culture from patient. • Test urine for haemoglobinuria. Complete and take to BB **Investigation of Suspected Trans. Reaction Form.**

Blood Bank 2422/2423. Out of hours bleep 267   **Blood Transfusion Nurse Specialist** ext. 4683 or Pager KH4683

If products are collected and **not used** they must be returned to the blood bank fridge within 30 minutes. After that please write on the back of the tag an explanation for the **wastage** and return the product to Blood Bank.
All adverse incidents are investigated & reported to: Hospital Transfusion Committee and Clinical Risk Management Group.
Certain blood transfusion events, reactions & Near Misses are reported nationally to MHRA and / or SHOT.

(b)

Figure 3.1b A summary of the procedure for the collection and administration of the blood and instructions in case of a transfusion reaction.

Table 3.1 Measures to avoid sampling errors.

• Tubes with blood samples must be clearly labelled with the patient's full name, hospital number and date of birth. Pre-printed labels ('addressographs') are not recommended in the UK, as they may be misfiled in the notes
• One patient should be bled at a time; tubes should be labelled after they are filled with blood
• The person who takes the blood must positively identify the patient by checking the wristband, and whenever possible, speaking to the patient
• No discrepancies are allowed between the information on the request form and on the tubes
• For patients with historical blood records current information must be identical with previous ones (the exception is for patients after haemopoietic stem cell transplantation)

Table 3.2 The ABO blood group system.

	Blood groups			
	O	**A**	**B**	**AB**
Antigens on red (and other) cells	None	A	B	A + B
Antibody in serum	Anti-AB	Anti-B	Anti-A	None
Approximate percentage in UK	47	42	8	3

(3–5 minutes) at room temperature ('immediate spin'). A second reason for crossmatching by IAT at 37°C is to detect an antibody against a low/moderate incidence antigen that may be present on donor cells but not on the screening cells (e.g. Wr^a, Js^a, C^w or antibodies against subgroups of A and B antigens, e.g. anti-A_1).

Is it necessary to perform all these tests? Studies conducted in the 1980s showed that if the crossmatch by IAT is omitted, the risk of missing an alloantibody is about one in 5500 samples. However, the risk of selecting an incompatible unit is between one in 10 000 and 50 000, depending on the frequency of the (missed) antibody and its antigen. Finally, a review of 1.3 million negative antibody screens and 'immediate spin' crossmatches in 20 US hospitals

Crossmatching

Crossmatching means testing the red cells from the donor units against the patient's plasma (or serum). If blood grouping has been carried out, and the antibody screen found negative, the main purpose of crossmatching is to confirm the ABO compatibility between the donor and the recipient. This can be done by a quick test

Table 3.3 Frequency (as percentage) of population positive for some red cell antigens in various racial groups.

Antigen	White Caucasian	Black African	Oriental
D	85	94	>99
K	9	1–2	0.02
Jk(b)	74	49	–
B	9–11	25–30	29

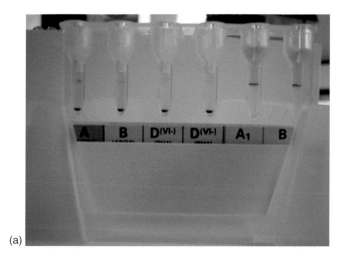

(a)

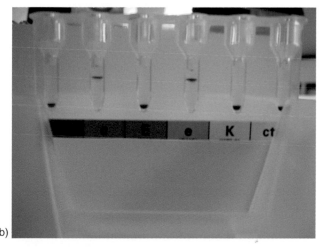

(b)

Figure 3.2 Gel column agglutination. The cells at the top of the column denote a positive result and those at the bottom a negative result. (a) Negative reactions with anti-A (blue), anti-B (yellow) and two anti-Ds indicate blood group O, RhD negative. Reverse typing (pink) confirms group O, showing positive reaction with A1 and B cells due to the presence of anti-A and anti-B in the patient's plasma. (b) A positive reaction with anti-c and anti-e, and negative with anti-C, anti-E and anti-K, shows the patient is group O, cde/cde (rr), K negative.

revealed only five haemolytic transfusion reactions, i.e. one in 260 000 crossmatches.

These findings have simplified pre-transfusion testing, and have led to the concept of the 'electronic' crossmatch (ElXm). Implementation of ElXm requires, in addition to reliable grouping and screening procedures, robust and safe blood ordering policies and reliable hospital computer systems. To be certain of the patient's ABO group, it is mandatory to test the patient on *at least two occasions* before blood is issued. Testing two separate samples ensures the presence of a 'historical group' on the blood bank computer system, which is paramount for blood safety. Performing two tests on a single sample eliminates laboratory error, but not the more common 'wrong blood in tube' situation.

If clinically significant antibodies are detected red cells negative for the corresponding antigen(s) should be selected, and a full serological crossmatch by IAT before transfusion will be needed on all occasions.

From the blood bank to the patient

Once blood is issued from the blood bank, it is labelled and assigned for an individual patient (the exception is the O RhD-negative blood kept for use in ungrouped patients with life-threatening bleeding, the 'flying squad' blood). The final step in the transfusion chain is the check, preferably performed by two people or with electronic aids, at the bedside or in the operating theatre, that the information on the compatibility form and the labels on the units of blood matches that on the transfusion prescription form, the patient's notes and the patient's wristband. Whenever possible the patient should be positively identified. The checking procedure, if not computerized, must be documented and signed by the two people concerned. In case of any doubt transfusion must be withheld until the discrepancy is resolved. The compatibility form, containing the donation numbers, blood groups, expiry dates of the units transfused, and signatures of the person(s) who conducted the check should be filed in the patient's notes. This is to ensure that the ultimate destination of each unit of blood is known, as required by law in the countries of the European Union. In this manner, if an adverse reaction occurs, the transfusion service will have no difficulty in tracing the donor. Increasingly, the compatibility form is being replaced by a unit tag with a peel-off label that contains the same set of data, and which can be stuck onto the transfusion prescription form, or in a designated place in the patient's notes. Although currently not widely used due to significant costs, computerized systems for patient/blood unit identification offer additional safety and will probably become the norm in the future.

Ordering blood for surgical operations

A large number of blood units are crossmatched for patients about to undergo elective surgery. Many of them will not be transfused, although compatible units of blood will have been reserved and kept unused during the perioperative period. Minimizing overordering is important, as it increases the available blood stock, and reduces wastage and the workload in the blood bank. For this reason, it is advisable that every hospital should analyse its usage of blood and establish the crossmatch to transfusion ratio for common elective surgery. If the ratio is more than 2:1 it is considered that an excessive number of units are being crossmatched for that type of operation.

Table 3.4 An example of a maximum surgical blood ordering schedule (MSBOS).

Cholecystectomy	G&S (group & save)
Hernia repair	G&S
Caesarean section	G&S
Hemicolectomy	G&S
Laparoscopy	G&S
Splenectomy	2 units
Coronary artery bypass	2 units
Radical prostatectomy	2–3 units
Aortofemoral bypass	6 units

After the crossmatch to transfusion ratios have been compiled, all those concerned (surgeons, anaesthetists, physicians and haematologists) should agree a list of common operations for which blood should be crossmatched, with the number of units to be crossmatched for each operation. Procedures for which less than 30% of patients require blood do not need to have blood crossmatched, and are listed as 'group and screen' operations. As an example, an audit at King's College Hospital, London, found that 27% of patients undergoing primary unilateral hip replacement were transfused. While crossmatching 2 units of blood was previously routinely requested for this operation, it has since been converted to 'group and screen'. The use of such a plan, particular to each hospital – referred to as the maximum surgical blood ordering schedule (MSBOS) (Table 3.4) – minimizes unnecessary crossmatching and helps the hospital to concentrate on providing blood for patients who really need it. These policies must not be rigid, and should be overruled if a patient is likely to need more blood than is stipulated, for example if the operation is expected to be more difficult than usual, or if the patient has a coagulation defect that is not readily correctable.

If the patient is found to have clinically significant alloantibodies, antigen-negative blood should be obtained, crossmatched and reserved, even when chances that transfusion will be needed are small. The surgeon and anaesthetist should be warned that, if the antigen-negative blood is difficult to find, it may be necessary to postpone the operation. This emphasizes the need for pre-transfusion testing to be done in pre-assessment clinics, well before admission for surgery.

In recent years there has been a trend towards reducing the number of blood units ordered and to convert many operations to 'group and screen'. The reasons for this are several: lower triggers for red cell transfusion have been widely accepted; the widespread use of blood conservation methods, like cell salvage; and novel techniques that reduce blood loss (e.g. 'off-pump' coronary artery bypass, see Chapter 16). Finally, EIXm allows the issue of group-specific blood within 10–15 minutes, even if this includes another ABO group check by the 'immediate spin' test. Conceivably, as the users' confidence in the blood bank's ability to supply blood grows, blood will need to be reserved only for a minority of operations, such as aortic aneurysm repair or orthotopic liver transplantation, where some blood will almost certainly be required in the course of surgery.

Adverse events

One of the main causes of serious morbidity and even mortality attributable to transfusion is human error. Errors can occur at every stage of the blood transfusion chain – when taking samples from the patient, during laboratory testing, at collection of blood from the blood bank, or during administration of the blood. As shown in Chapter 18, an alarming incidence of non-compliance with procedures is reported year on year, leading to incompatible transfusions, haemolytic transfusion reactions and, in a few cases, death. Hospital transfusion committees are responsible for monitoring, reporting and taking corrective action for adverse incidents of transfusion in hospitals.

Further reading

British Committee for Standards in Haematology, Blood Transfusion Task Force Guidelines for compatibility procedures in blood transfusion laboratories. *Transfusion Medicine* 2004; **14**: 59–73.

Emily Cooley Lecture 2002: transfusion safety in the hospital. *Transfusion* 2003; **43**: 1190–9.

Goodnough LT, Shander A, Brecher ME. Transfusion medicine: looking to the future. *Lancet* 2003; **361**: 161–9.

McCullough J. *Transfusion Medicine*, 2nd edn. Elsevier/Churchill Livingstone, London, 2005.

Mollison PL, Engelfriet CP, Contreras M. *Blood Transfusion in Clinical Medicine*, 10th edn. Blackwell Publishing, Oxford, 1997.

CHAPTER 4

Red Cell Transfusion

Mike Murphy and Jonathan Wallis

OVERVIEW

- Red cell transfusion is given to increase oxygen delivery from the lungs to tissues and in particular to the myocardium.
- A postoperative transfusion threshold of 7–8 g/dl is suitable for healthy adults.
- A postoperative threshold of 8–9 g/dl is suitable for patients with known cardiovascular disease.
- Pre-transfusion checks *must* be carried out at the bedside.
- In an emergency, uncrossmatched O RhD-negative blood is safe to transfuse in >99% of patients.

This chapter considers the red cell preparations currently available, the indications for their use, their administration, and potential harmful effects. Use of red cell concentrates has fallen by about 15% in the last 5 years in England, largely due to acceptance of lower transfusion triggers in elective surgery. This change in practice has been due to concerns about the risks of transfusion, the cost of transfusion and developments of alternatives such as red cell salvage. These issues are described in more detail elsewhere in the book.

Recipients of red cell transfusions

In the UK most blood goes to older patients (median age of 65 years) (Figure 4.1). Only about 33% is now given for surgical indications. Haematological disease and gastrointestinal haemorrhage are the leading medical indications (Figure 4.2).

Preparation of red cells

Each unit of red cells comes from a single donation of 470 ml (range 405–495 ml) whole blood taken into citrate anticoagulant, and contains >40 g haemoglobin (Hb) per unit (Figure 4.3). In the UK all red cell units originating from whole blood are filtered to remove >99.9% of white cells, leaving <5 × 10^6 leucocytes per unit. Filtration also removes all the platelets.

The collection of 2 units of red cells from donors with large blood volumes, by apheresis, at a single session is being piloted by the National Blood Service and may become more widespread with time.

Red cells in saline adenine glucose mannitol (SAG-M) are processed by the removal of >90% of the plasma and resuspension of the red cells in an approved additive solution made up of saline, adenine, glucose and mannitol for optimal red cell storage (final volume 280 ± 60 ml) (Figure 4.4). This is the standard product in the UK.

About 5% of units simply have some of the plasma removed to give plasma reduced cells with a similar final volume. Washed red cells are prepared to remove nearly all the plasma (residual protein <0.5 g/unit) for specific patients with adverse reactions to plasma proteins or to remove anti-A or anti-B for mismatched solid organ transplants. Frozen and thawed red cells allow for the storage of rare donor or autologous red cells for patients with single or multiple red cell antibodies that make the provision of matched donor blood difficult. Frozen units can be stored for up to 10 years.

Storage of red cell units

Red cell units are stored at 4 ± 2°C, both to preserve red cell function by reducing red cell metabolic requirements and to prevent bacterial growth from any chance contaminants. During storage intracellular potassium leaks out of red cells. Levels of extracellular K$^+$ rise to as much as 50 mmol/L by 35 days (more rapidly in irradiated units) but as the extracellular fluid volume is small the total K$^+$ load is usually <5 mmol (Table 4.1). Intracellular energy supplies in the form of adenosine triphosphate (ATP) are reduced by about 50%, and 2,3-diphosphoglycerate (2,3-DPG), an intermediary in the glycolytic pathway, falls to near zero after 9 days. Membrane changes also occur with a reduction in deformability and there is some loss of lipid and protein as microvesicles. These membrane changes are partly or largely reversible and are less pronounced in leucocyte-depleted units.

After transfusion the red cell ATP level rises to above normal levels within 1 hour but the 2,3-DPG level rises more slowly. The 2,3-DPG concentration is one of the factors controlling the Hb oxygen affinity curve. A low 2,3-DPG level significantly increases the oxygen affinity of Hb and leads to less oxygen off-loading in tissues. The recovery of 2,3-DPG after transfusion is shown in

ABC of Transfusion, 4th edition, 2009. Edited by Marcela Contreras. © 2009 Blackwell Publishing, ISBN: 978-1-4051-5646-2.

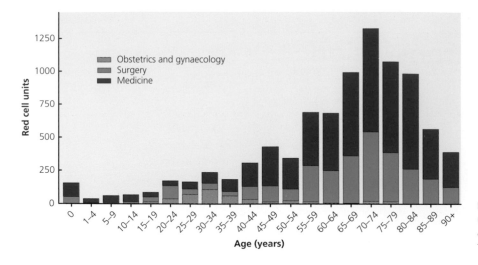

Figure 4.1 Age distribution of transfusion recipients in the north of England in 2004, according to the specialty under which they were transfused.

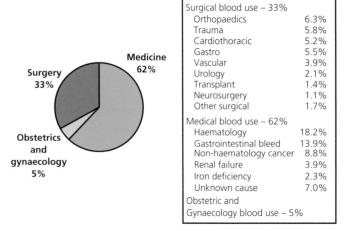

Surgical blood use – 33%	
Orthopaedics	6.3%
Trauma	5.8%
Cardiothoracic	5.2%
Gastro	5.5%
Vascular	3.9%
Urology	2.1%
Transplant	1.4%
Neurosurgery	1.1%
Other surgical	1.7%
Medical blood use – 62%	
Haematology	18.2%
Gastrointestinal bleed	13.9%
Non-haematology cancer	8.8%
Renal failure	3.9%
Iron deficiency	2.3%
Unknown cause	7.0%
Obstetric and Gynaecology blood use – 5%	

Figure 4.2 Use of red cells in the north of England in 2004.

Figure 4.5. Even the moderate reduction in 2,3-DPG that persists at 24 hours after transfusion is sufficient in theory to have an adverse effect on oxygen delivery to tissues (Figure 4.6). However, there is little hard evidence for or against a clinically significant effect. The red cell membrane defects acquired on storage are of uncertain clinical significance.

In the UK, red cells are stored for up to 35 days before transfusion. This time limit is based on a required viability of 75% of transfused red cells 24 hours after transfusion. Leucocyte-depleted red cells in additive solution perform much better than this, with ≥90% survival 24 hours post-transfusion after 35 days storage.

Rationale for the use of red cell transfusions

The only true indication for red cell transfusions is a need to rapidly increase the delivery of oxygen to the tissues. The heart extracts 60–70% of oxygen from the blood flowing through the coronary arteries (the next most oxygen-hungry organ, other than exercising skeletal muscle, is the brain, which takes about 30% of the oxygen from perfusing blood). Because the heart is already

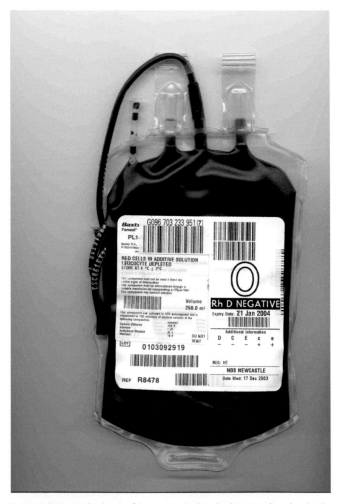

Figure 4.3 A standard unit of leucocyte-depleted, plasma-reduced red cells resuspended in optimal additive solution.

off-loading the majority of oxygen from red cells in normal circumstances, both increased cardiac output (increased cardiac work) and anaemia require an increase in coronary blood flow to supply adequate oxygen to the myocardium. Healthy coronary arteries can dilate, and so increase blood flow, by as much as five-fold. Unhealthy or stenosed coronary arteries may not be able to do so. If the coronary blood flow fails to deliver sufficient oxygen the heart muscle becomes relatively hypoxic, and there will be a fall in cardiac output and a reduction in systemic blood flow that may lead to organ failure. Anaemia and coronary artery disease together place a particular stress on adequate myocardial oxygenation (Figure 4.7). Transfusion is therefore first and foremost to maintain oxygen delivery to the heart, which in turn will maintain perfusion and oxygen supply to other organs.

Effects of anaemia

Retrospective studies in Jehovah's Witnesses refusing transfusion have shown a marked rise in mortality and serious morbidity when the preoperative Hb is <5 g/dl. The relationship between mortality and preoperative Hb is shown in Figure 4.8, which emphasizes the finding that patients with pre-existing cardiovascular disease show a greater risk of death for the same degree of anaemia. Healthy, resting humans can tolerate a surprising degree of acute normovolaemic anaemia, but patients are not always healthy and often not at rest. Transfusion triggers or thresholds will differ depending on clinical circumstances. The situation in acute anaemia may be very different from that in chronic anaemia when patients will

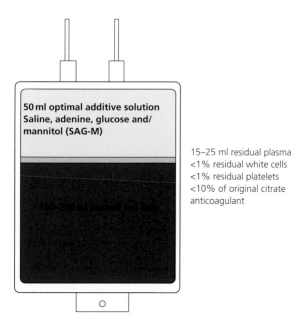

Figure 4.4 A schematic unit of red cells in SAG-M showing the typical contents.

50 ml optimal additive solution
Saline, adenine, glucose and/mannitol (SAG-M)

15–25 ml residual plasma
<1% residual white cells
<1% residual platelets
<10% of original citrate anticoagulant

often compensate well both physiologically and by modifying their lifestyle.

Appropriate transfusion thresholds for red cell transfusion

The following questions should be considered when deciding whether to transfuse red cells:
- Is the patient symptomatic?
- Is the anaemia acute or chronic?
- Is the patient likely to resume physical activities immediately or is he/she bedbound?
- Does the patient have a history of heart or respiratory disease?
- Is the patient septic or already in heart failure?
- Is the anaemia correctable with measures other than transfusion?

Postoperative transfusion triggers of an Hb level of 7–8 g/dl for healthy adults and children have become widely accepted and appear to be safe. In older and frailer patients or those with cardiovascular disease, a threshold of 8–9 g/dl is acceptable. Similar thresholds are appropriate in critically ill patients without active bleeding.

Patients who present with well-compensated anaemia due to correctable haematinic deficiencies will usually manage without transfusion unless they are markedly symptomatic. Patients with anaemia of chronic disease rarely require or benefit from transfusion.

Patients with bone marrow failure typically become symptomatic when the Hb falls below 9 g/dl. Transfusion thresholds vary between 7 and 10 g/dl in this group and should be based individually on symptoms. Patients with renal failure who are failing to respond to erythropoietin should be transfused as for bone marrow failure.

There is evidence that an Hb of >11 g/dl, even if achieved by transfusion, improves the response of cervical cancer to radiotherapy.

Administration of red cells

In patients with active bleeding, red cell units should be given as quickly as required to keep up with blood loss. In a chronically anaemic patient each unit of red cells can safely be given over 90 minutes, and 4 units given over 6 hours. The infusion rate should be adjusted appropriately for small adults or children. There is

Table 4.1 Potassium levels in red cells stored in additive solution (data compiled by M. Wiltshire and S. Thomas, National Blood Service).

	Day 0	Day 1	Day 7	Day 14	Day 21	Day 28	Day 35
Free K+(mmol/L)1	1.19 ± 0.23	1.40 ± 0.32	16.8 ± 6.57	26.9 ± 7.86	33.2 ± 6.23	40.5 ± 4.31	44.0 ± 8.12
Free K+ (mmol/unit)*	0.15 ± 0.2	0.18 ± 0.07	1.88 ± 0.60	2.88 ± 0.90	_	_	4.67 ± 0.95

Results are mean ± SD.
* n ≥ 20.

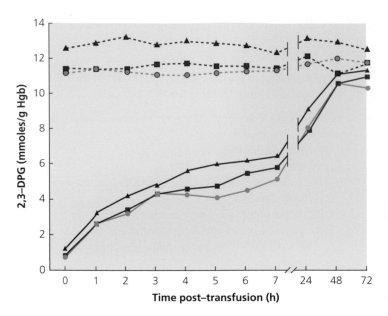

Figure 4.5 Recovery of 2,3-diphosphoglycerate (2,3-DPG) in transfused red cells. The three solid lines show the recovery of 2,3-DPG after the transfusion of red cells kept in three different storage media. The hashed lines show 2,3-DPG levels in the recipients' own cells. There is an early and rapid recovery of about 50% of normal 2,3-DPG at 6 hours after transfusion, 66% recovery by 24 hours, and essentially complete recovery at 48 hours. (Reproduced with permission from Heaton et al. 1989.)

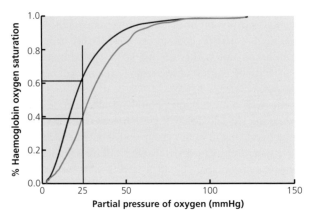

Figure 4.6 The haemoglobin–oxygen disassociation curve. A moderate reduction in red cell 2,3-DPG (blue curve) has a marked effect on oxygen unloading compared to normal (green curve). At a partial pressure of 25 mmHg oxygen, typical in the myocardium, oxygen unloading is reduced by a third from about 60% of bound oxygen to just 40%.

no need to use any routine premedication unless the patient has a history of:

- repeated febrile reactions; treat with oral paracetamol 1 g 6-hourly, and i.v. hydrocortisone 100 mg if severe
- recurrent urticaria associated with transfusion; treat with i.v. chlorpheniramine 10 mg 6-hourly
- heart failure; treat with frusemide 20–80 mg orally or intravenously depending on the dose of any regular diuretics. If the patient is in heart failure then the rate of transfusion may be slowed, or only 1 or 2 units transfused at a time with a gap for recovery before further transfusion.

Drugs and other fluids should never be mixed directly with the blood in the bag, and calcium-containing solutions or hypotonic solutions such as 5% dextrose should not be used to flush lines. Red cells should be administered using a standard drip set with a

170 μm mesh filter. Bedside leucocyte depletion filters are superfluous if all red cell units are already leucocyte depleted, as in the UK. Large volumes of blood and other fluids being administered rapidly should be warmed in a blood warmer at infusion to prevent hypothermia, which will worsen haemostasis.

Patients receiving red cell transfusions should be monitored by checking and recording pulse, blood pressure and temperature *before, at 15 minutes and after* every unit of blood. The patient should be observed particularly carefully for the first 15 minutes of each transfusion. If the patient is suspected of having a serious adverse event during a transfusion the transfusion should be stopped and appropriate investigations carried out.

Expected benefits of red cell transfusion

Normal red cells produced by the marrow have a lifespan of 110–120 days. Donor red cells are on average 60 days old when collected, therefore the lifespan of transfused red cells is on average 60 days. In a chronically anaemic adult, a typical 3 unit top-up transfusion will increase the Hb by 2–3 g/dl, say from 7 to 10 g/dl all told. In patients with little or no effective red cell production of their own, the Hb would fall to 7 g/dl again after 21 days. Chronically transfused patients typically report a delayed benefit that is most noticeable by the second day after transfusion. This may relate to the recovery of red cell 2,3-DPG with the enhanced oxygen offloading that this produces. Patients usually report 1 week, or at most 2 weeks, improved energy followed by increasing fatigue.

In patients with severe acute anaemia the beneficial effects of transfusion are immediate, and may be marked. In acute bleeding a haematocrit of >30% (approximate Hb of 10 g/dl) has been shown to be associated with a reduced skin bleeding time. It has been suggested that this is due to the peripheral partitioning of platelets by the axial flowing red cells within the blood vessels, so improving platelet–vessel wall interactions.

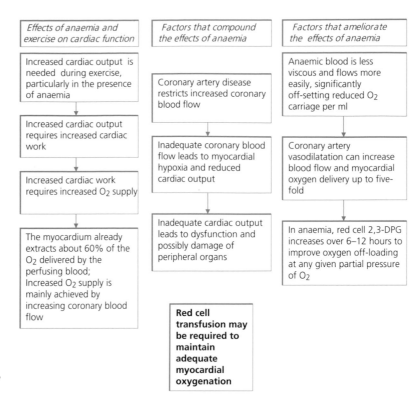

Figure 4.7 Anaemia, myocardial oxygenation and cardiac output. O_2, oxygen.

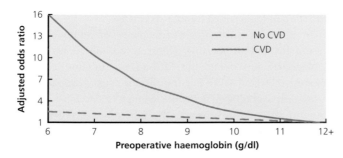

Figure 4.8 The odds ratio for death in Jehovah's Witnesses presenting for surgery according to the level of preoperative anaemia. The likelihood of death rose moderately with increasing anaemia for those patients without cardiovascular disease, but much more rapidly for those patients with anaemia and cardiovascular disease. (Reproduced with permission from Carson et al. 1996.)

Adverse effects of red cell transfusions

The UK haemovigilance scheme, Serious Hazards of Transfusion (SHOT), collects reports of adverse transfusion events (see Chapter 15). ABO incompatible red cell transfusion remains one of the most important serious hazards of transfusion and is a much greater risk than that of human immunodeficiency virus (HIV) or hepatitis C virus (HCV) transmission by blood (Figure 4.9). Box 4.1 provides learning points for the avoidance of transfusion errors collated from the SHOT annual report for 2003. The following risks are those most often encountered in the UK:

1 *ABO incompatible transfusions* usually, though not always, produce immediate intravascular haemolysis with pain at the site of infusion, an initial increase in blood pressure, loin pain and haemoglobinuria, followed, in about 10–20% of patients, by hypotensive shock, disseminated intravascular coagulation (DIC) and renal failure. Fortunately, serious haemolytic transfusion reactions due to ABO incompatible transfusions are rare occurrences (around one in 100 000 transfused units), but several deaths are reported each year in the UK. They are due to errors at some stage in the transfusion process, such as collection of the blood sample for compatibility testing from the wrong patient or labelling it with the wrong patient's identification details; technical and sample handling errors in the laboratory; collection of the wrong blood from the blood refrigerator; and administration of the blood to the wrong patient. Rapid recognition, diagnosis and prompt treatment are vital. If a severe transfusion reaction is suspected the transfusion should be stopped immediately; the blood unit and a new blood sample should be sent to the laboratory for urgent investigation.

2 *Acute haemolytic reactions* due to other red cell antibodies are rarer but may be missed if not considered. Delayed haemolytic reactions due to atypical red cell antibodies develop 3 days to 3 weeks after transfusion, and occasionally result in symptomatic extravascular haemolysis.

3 *Non-haemolytic febrile transfusion reactions* remain common, although they have decreased significantly following universal leucodepletion (one in 500 transfused units), but are rarely clinically important.

4 *Urticaria* is a minor reaction and does not necessitate stopping of the transfusion unless it is part of anaphylaxis or a severe general allergic reaction.

5 *Bacterial infected units* causing acute shock are very rare but should always be considered when a severe, early transfusion

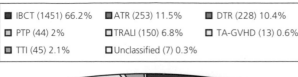
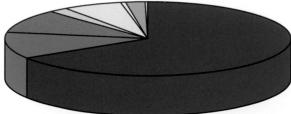

Figure 4.9 A total of 2191 cumulative incidents from the UK reported to SHOT between 1996 and 2003 show that incorrect blood transfusion remains the most common transfusion error. ATR, acute transfusion reaction; DTR, delayed transfusion reaction; IBCT, incorrect blood component transfused; PTP, post-transfusion purpura; TA-GvHD, transfusion-associated graft-versus-host disease; TRALI, transfusion-related acute lung injury; and TTI, transfusion-transmitted infection.

Box 4.1 **Learning points for the avoidance of transfusion errors collated from the Serious Hazards of Transfusion (SHOT) annual report 2003**

- The final patient identity check prior to transfusion must be done at the bedside against an identification wristband or equivalent attached to the patient (Figure 4.10).
- Mislabelling of patient samples can result in potentially fatal ABO incompatible transfusion. Samples should be labelled at the bedside.
- A decision to transfuse must take account of clinical as well as laboratory results; unexpected laboratory results should be confirmed.
- Errors occur more often when staff are under pressure and there is a high level of stress, both at the bedside and in the laboratory. Safety must not be compromised in emergency situations.
- Laboratory staff working out of hours and/or under pressure must be supported by robust procedures and technology, and should not be required to work beyond their level of competence or experience.
- Transfusion laboratory information technology systems should alert staff to select appropriate blood components.
- Patients should be educated regarding their special requirements and staff should take note of information from patients.
- Education and training are of key importance for safe and effective transfusion practice.

reaction occurs. Blood samples from the patient and the blood unit should be sent for culture.

6 *Acute transfusion-related acute lung injury* (TRALI) is uncommon with red cells in additive solution or plasma-reduced red cells transfused slowly, but may occur during rapid infusion for bleeding. This type of reaction should be suspected when there is acute-onset pulmonary oedema, especially with hypotension and frothy tracheal aspirate.

7 *Volume overload* with cardiogenic pulmonary oedema is not common with red cell transfusions, but may be difficult to distinguish from TRALI acutely.

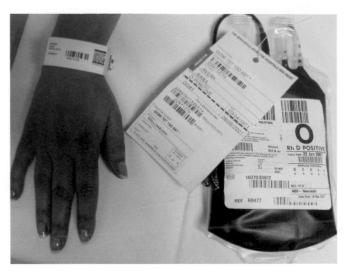

Figure 4.10 Bedside administration errors are the most common cause of an ABO incompatible transfusion. Be sure to check the patient identity, both verbally and from the wristband, with the patient details on the compatibility label attached to the unit of blood, and a record in the notes according to local protocols.

8 *Immunomodulation.* There is no convincing evidence that leucocyte-depleted red cell transfusion has any significant immunomodulatory effect leading either to an increased risk of infection or to increased tumour recurrence.

9 *Iron overload* is an inevitable consequence of continued transfusion for chronic marrow failure or haemolysis or haemoglobinopathies without the lifelong use of iron chelation treatment (Figure 4.11). For transfusion-dependent patients in whom survival is likely to be long enough to develop complications of iron overload chelation must be considered. For young patients with haemoglobinopathies or haemolysis, it should be planned in good time by the specialist centre responsible for their care. In older patients with aplastic anaemia or myelodysplasia the decision to start iron chelation depends on prognosis and acceptability. Iron chelation should be given active consideration after the transfusion of a total of 40 units of red cells.

10 *Alloantibodies to red cells* may develop in the chronically transfused. Multiple antibodies can make the provision of compatible red cells difficult. There is some evidence that routine matching for antigens such as Rh Cc/Ee (in addition to D) and Kell reduces immunization to other antigens. It is recommended that such matching is done for haemoglobinopathy patients, and some consider that it should be done for all chronically transfused patients.

Red cell transfusion in an emergency

Patients with acute bleeding in whom the blood group and antibody screen results are not yet available can be transfused with group O Rh-negative blood. Very rarely (less than one in 200) the patient will have an atypical red cell alloantibody (e.g. anti-c) that will react with O RhD-negative blood. If the patient has an antibody card or is known to have antibodies, discuss urgently with

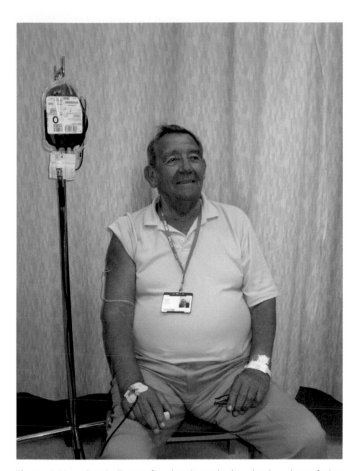

Figure 4.11 A chronically transfused patient who has developed transfusion associated haemosiderosis. Note the greyish all-over tan due to iron deposition in the skin, and the subcutaneous needle in the right shoulder for infusion of the iron chelator, desferrrioxamine. The patient photo ID card is being used to check patient identity.

the laboratory but do not withhold transfusion for life-threatening bleeding. As soon as the patient's blood group is known, red cells of the same ABO and Rh group may be given. In the case of male patients and women past childbearing age with no preformed anti-D, even if they are group O RhD-negative, group O RhD-positive red cells can be transfused safely. This policy will avoid depletion of stocks of group O Rh-negative red cells.

Further reading

British Committee for Standards in Haematology. Guidelines for the administration of blood components and the management of transfused patients. *Transfusion Medicine* 1999; **9**: 227–38.

British Committee for Standards in Haematology. Guidelines for the clinical use of red cell transfusion. *British Journal of Haematology* 2001; **113**: 24–31.

Carson JL, Duff A, Poses RM, Berlin JA, Spence RK, Trout R, Noveck H, Strom BL. Effect of anaemia and cardiovascular disease on surgical mortality and morbidity. *Lancet* 1996; **348**: 1055–60.

Heaton A, Keegan T, Home S. In vivo regeneration of red cell 2,3diphosphoglycerate following transfusion of DPG-depleted AS-1, AS-3 and CPD-1 red cells. *British Journal of Haematology* 1989; **71**; 131–6.

Hébert PC, Wells G, Blajchman MA, et al. A multicenter, randomized, controlled clinical trial of transfusion requirements in critical care. *New England Journal of Medicine* 1999; **340**: 409–17.

Serious Hazards of Transfusion (SHOT) scheme. *Annual Report 2003*. SHOT, Manchester, 2006, www.shotuk.org.

CHAPTER 5

Platelet and Granulocyte Transfusions

Modupe Elebute, Simon Stanworth and Cristina Navarrete

OVERVIEW

- Platelet transfusions are invaluable for the prevention or treatment of life-threatening bleeding in patients with severe thrombocytopenia and in patients with inherited disorders of platelet function.

- Platelet transfusions are ineffective in acquired platelet dysfunction and in autoimmune thrombocytopenic purpura but may be given to support life-threatening bleeding in these patients.

- Platelet transfusions are contraindicated in patients with thrombotic thrombocytopenic purpura, haemolytic uraemic syndrome or heparin-induced thrombocytopenia.

- A major, potentially fatal, risk of platelet transfusions is acute haemolytic transfusion reaction due to bacterial contamination because platelets are stored at room temperature, facilitating bacterial growth.

- There has been renewed interest in the use of granulocyte transfusions to support patients with prolonged neutropenia with serious infections.

- Potentially serious adverse effects and lack of efficacy of granulocyte transfusions in the published literature limit their use to desperately ill patients with bacterial or fungal sepsis resulting from prolonged neutropenia.

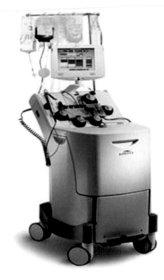

Figure 5.1 Centrifugation blood cell separator machine (Trima® Accel™ Collection System) (courtesy of GAMBRO BCT).

Platelet transfusions are used for the treatment or prevention of life-threatening bleeding in patients with severe thrombocytopenia, most often caused by bone marrow failure. Thrombocytopenia may be the direct consequence of bone marrow infiltration (for example, acute leukaemia), of bone marrow failure due to disease (aplastic anaemia) or of treatment with cytotoxic agents. Platelet transfusions have made potentially curative intensive cytotoxic treatment regimens, with or without stem cell transplantation, possible.

Interest in the use of granulocyte transfusions has been renewed due to the increase in numbers of patients with (or at high risk of) fungal infections arising from periods of prolonged neutropenia following more intensive chemotherapy regimens. Granulocyte transfusions also appear to be beneficial in patients with life-threatening infection and disorders of abnormal neutrophil function. The development of centrifugation cell separators and the availability of granulocyte colony-stimulating factor (G-CSF) has made possible the collection of greater numbers of granulocytes from donors. There is, however, little published literature on the clinical efficacy of transfused granulocytes and well recognized potentially serious complications.

Preparation of platelet and granulocyte concentrates

Platelet concentrates can be prepared from units of blood collected from random donors into multiple blood collection packs or, alternatively, a cell separator (apheresis machine; Figure 5.1) can be used to collect platelets from a single donor. In the United Kingdom all red cell and platelet concentrates have been leucodepleted since 1999 (see Chapter 14).

The properties of the different platelet concentrates available in the UK are outlined in Table 5.1. Platelets should be kept agitated at $22 \pm 2°C$ and have a shelf life of 5 days, although this can be extended to 7 days with appropriate bacteriological monitoring.

ABC of Transfusion, 4th edition, 2009. Edited by Marcela Contreras. © 2009 Blackwell Publishing, ISBN: 978-1-4051-5646-2.

Table 5.1 Properties of platelet concentrates (from McClelland 2007).

	Platelets, buffy coat derived, leucocyte depleted (random donor)	Platelets, apheresis, leucocyte depleted (single donor)	HLA/HPA typed apheresis platelets (see Chapter 11)	Crossmatched apheresis platelets (see Chapter 11)
Unit	A pool derived from four buffy coats	One (adult) donation		
Volume*	Up to 300 ml of plasma from one of the donors involved	Mean 215 ml (range 180–300 ml) Check local product specification		
Content of platelets	$\geq240 \times 10^9$ per pool	$\geq240 \times 10^9$ per unit (one donation may contain 2 units)		
Content of white cells	$<5 \times 10^6$	$<5 \times 10^6$		
Adult dose	One pool	One unit		
Points to note when prescribing	Contain sufficient volume (200–300 ml) of a single donor's plasma to cause haemolysis if the donor has potent ABO antibodies. Donor should be ABO compatible for plasma and cells			

* Typical volumes are given.

Table 5.2 Properties of different granulocyte concentrates (data provided by Rebecca Cardigan, Saber Bashir and Fred Goddard, Component Development Laboratory, NHSBT, UK).

	Single buffy coat ($n = 21$) (mean, SD)	10 buffy coats (dose typically transfused for adults)	Unstimulated apheresis collection ($n = 20$) (mean, SD)	Stimulated apheresis collection ($n = 5$) (median, range)
Volume (ml)	59 (3)	590	279 (46)	299 (214–333)
Neutrophils (10^{10}/U)	0.105 (0.04)	1.05	0.54 (0.2)	6.37 (3.69–8.47)
Haematocrit (%)	45 (6)	45	23 (7)	9 (7–20)
Platelets (10^9/U)	70 (22)	700	111 (25)	160 (82–293)
Red cells (10^{12}/U)	0.27 (0.04)	2.70	0.71 (0.23)	3 (2.8–6.1)

Granulocyte concentrates can be harvested as buffy coats prepared from 10 whole blood donations or by apheresis, either from unstimulated donors or from donors who have received corticosteroids and/or G-CSF shortly before the procedure. The properties of the different granulocyte concentrates available in the UK are outlined in Table 5.2. Granulocytes should be kept without agitation at 22 ± 2°C and transfused as soon as possible after collection/preparation; the product has a 24-hour expiry shelf life. Recent work in the UK has evaluated a different technique for the preparation of granulocytes derived from whole blood, and this may represent an improvement on the existing buffy coat component.

In special circumstances there is a need for platelet concentrates to be collected from donors whose human leucocyte antigen (HLA) or human platelet antigen (HPA, platelet-specific) phenotype is compatible with the patient's antibodies (see Chapter 11).

Platelet transfusions

Indications for platelet transfusions

Platelet transfusions (Figure 5.2) may be used prophylactically to prevent bleeding in thrombocytopenic patients or therapeutically to stop haemorrhage. In the UK most platelet concentrates are

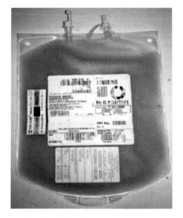

Figure 5.2 Leucocyte-depleted platelet concentrate.

transfused prophylactically; the following are the major indications for platelet transfusion:

Bone marrow failure caused by disease, myelosuppressive treatment or following haematopoietic stem cell transplantation

Severe bleeding in patients with bone marrow failure resulting from disease or caused by treatment may be prevented by maintaining

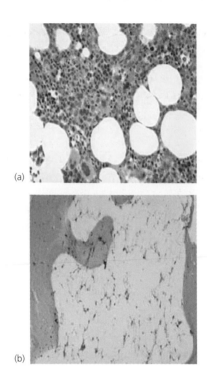

(a)

(b)

Figure 5.3 Bone marrow trephine biopsy showing (a) the normal ratio of haemopoietic cells and fat spaces, and (b) a lack of haemopoietic cells in aplastic anaemia.

the platelet count above 10×10^9/L. Figure 5.3 shows the architecture of a normal bone marrow biopsy and a marrow in aplastic anaemia. An increased dose and frequency of transfusions may be required to support patients with increased platelet consumption due to haemorrhage, febrile episodes, abnormal coagulation (as in disseminated intravascular coagulopathy, DIC) or splenomegaly.

Abnormalities of platelet function

Platelet transfusions are indicated in patients with inherited disorders of platelet function (e.g. Glanzmann's thrombasthenia, Bernard–Soulier syndrome and platelet storage pool deficiency) who develop serious haemorrhage or who require surgery. Platelet transfusions are ineffective in secondary or acquired platelet dysfunction due to myeloma, paraproteinaemia and uraemia. Abnormal platelet function caused by drugs (e.g. aspirin) may be irreversible until sufficient unexposed new platelets have been formed, or may improve rapidly once the drug is discontinued (e.g. non-steroidal anti-inflammatory analgesics).

Dilutional thrombocytopenia

Thrombocytopenia due to massive or exchange transfusions should be treated with platelet concentrates if the platelet count is less than 50×10^9/L and the patient is bleeding. The threshold may be higher in special circumstances such as intracranial bleeding, neurosurgery or in newborn infants.

Cardiopulmonary bypass surgery

Platelet transfusions are not indicated routinely in cardiac surgery. Haemorrhage during or after cardiopulmonary bypass may be caused by dilutional thrombocytopenia or by damage to platelets in the extracorporeal circulation. Platelet transfusions are helpful in both these situations. If possible all antiplatelet agents including aspirin and clopidogrel should be discontinued, or replaced by alternatives, at least 10 days before surgery to decrease the risk of bleeding.

Autoimmune thrombocytopenic purpura

Transfused platelets are destroyed by circulating autoantibodies in this condition and are therefore ineffective. However, platelet transfusions are given to support life-threatening bleeding in patients with severe, refractory autoimmune thrombocytopenic purpura.

Alloimmune thrombocytopenia

Maternal alloimmunization to paternal HPA is one of the main causes of thrombocytopenia in the newborn. Similarly, preformed HPA alloantibodies in adults can result in severe thrombocytopenia when transfused with blood components expressing the relevant antigen. In these cases transfusions with appropriate HPA-negative platelets may be indicated, either as prophylaxis or in the face of active bleeding

Administration of platelet concentrates

Platelet concentrates should be transfused over 30 minutes through a fresh platelet or standard blood administration set. One adult dose is equivalent either to one apheresis pack or to one buffy coat-derived platelet pool (see Figure 5.2); the paediatric dose is 10–15 ml/kg. ABO and RhD identical units should be used as far as is possible. To prevent acute haemolysis group O platelets should not be used, or used only as a last resort, for groups A, B or AB patients. In emergencies, group O platelets may be used for non-O recipients if the units have been tested and labelled as negative for high titre anti-A and anti-B. RhD-negative subjects given RhD-positive platelets may very rarely develop anti-D through sensitization by red cells present in the platelet concentrate. In girls and women of childbearing age this can be prevented by subcutaneous administration of 250 IU of anti-D immunoglobulin. Gamma-irradiated platelet concentrates should be given to immunocompromised patients, including all patients with Hodgkin's disease, and to recipients of HLA-matched platelets and of platelet concentrates collected from first degree relatives, in order to prevent transfusion-associated graft-versus-host disease (TA-GvHD) (see Chapter 11).

Platelet recovery

The expected recovery of platelets 1 hour after transfusion is 50–80% and their half-life in the circulation is about 4 days. The efficacy of each platelet transfusion should be checked by clinical observation, by monitoring the platelet count increment (either at 24 hours or at 1 hour) and, in some cases, by calculating the corrected platelet increment (referenced in many general textbooks of transfusion). In a clinically stable patient, the expected increment after one dose of platelets is $30–40 \times 10^9$/L.

Indications for antigen-matched or crossmatch compatible platelet transfusions

Immunological refractoriness to platelet transfusions

Immunological refractoriness may be defined as the failure of two consecutive ABO identical, fresh platelet transfusions to give a corrected increment of $>7.5 \times 10^9$/L 1 hour after transfusion in the absence of fever, severe haemorrhage, splenomegaly or DIC. Refractoriness is caused by alloantibodies to HLA and, rarely, to platelet-specific antigens, stimulated by previous transfusion or pregnancy. Although 30–70% of recipients of multiple transfusions of platelet concentrates from random donors become alloimmunized to HLA, only some will become immunologically 'refractory'. The presence of antibodies to HLA in the patient's serum should be confirmed. If necessary, the presence of anti-HPA should be investigated. HLA-matched or crossmatch compatible platelets are required for future support of immunologically refractory patients with confirmed HLA- or HPA-specific antibodies.

Bleeding in patients who lack human platelet antigens

Patients who lack the glycoproteins carrying HPAs, such as those with Glanzmann's thrombasthenia or Bernard–Soulier syndrome, may develop isoantibodies after transfusion or pregnancy. The current protocol for the transfusion support of such patients includes the use of HLA-matched platelets on the assumption that these will reduce the risk of alloimmunization in these transfusion-dependent patients.

Patients with preformed anti-HPA can develop post-transfusion purpura (PTP) when challenged by subsequent transfusions of blood components that contain platelets. Most PTP reactions are due to the presence of anti-HPA-1a, but antibodies against other HPA specificities have also been responsible. The current treatment of choice for these patients is the use of intravenous immunoglobulin (2 g/kg over 2–5 consecutive days). Transfusions of random or antigen-matched platelets are not very effective.

HPA-1a positive fetuses and infants of HPA-1a negative mothers with anti-HPA-1a may develop severe neonatal alloimmune thrombocytopenia (NAIT) following transplacental transfer of the antibody. Although anti-HPA-1a, and to a lesser extent anti-HPA-5b, are the main antibody specificities involved, antibodies against other HPA specificities have also been described. Similarly to the case of PTP, antibodies to other HPAs have also been found to be involved. HPA-1a (or the relevant antigen) negative platelets should be used for the treatment of thrombocytopenic patients with anti-HPA-1a and for fetuses and infants affected by NAIT due to anti-HPA-1a. If HPA-negative platelets are not available or in an emergency, random, ABO compatible platelet concentrates should be transfused.

Adverse effects of platelet transfusions

Most of the adverse effects common to other blood components may also occur following platelet transfusions (see Chapters 11–13). The most common adverse effect of platelet transfusion is the development of immunological reactions such as non-haemolytic febrile transfusion reactions (NHFTRs). Febrile reactions can be caused by white cell antibodies, mainly HLAs, present in the recipient and reacting with donor leucocytes, or, rarely, by interleukins and tumour necrosis factor released by leucocytes present in the platelet concentrate during storage. Other adverse effects are platelet refractoriness, TA-GvHD and allergic or anaphylactic reactions to plasma proteins such as immunoglobulin A (see Chapter 11). In addition the possible transmission of viruses, bacteria and prions remains a serious risk for all transfusions of blood components.

Cytomegalovirus (CMV) persists in the leucocytes of some of the individuals who have had an infection in the past. Transmission of CMV by transfusion to immunocompromised recipients may cause a severe and sometimes fatal infection. Therefore, transfusion of platelets collected from CMV-negative donors or knowingly leucodepleted platelet concentrates are indicated for these patients.

Bacterial contamination and endotoxic transmission are major risks of platelet transfusions because platelets are stored at room temperature, facilitating bacterial growth. Most of the cases of transfusion-transmitted bacterial infection reported to various haemovigilance programmes are caused by platelet transfusions.

Contraindications to platelet transfusions

Platelet transfusions should not be given to patients with thrombotic thrombocytopenic purpura, haemolytic uraemic syndrome or heparin-induced thrombocytopenia.

Granulocyte transfusions

Indications for granulocyte transfusions

Bone marrow failure caused by disease or myelotoxic treatment

Granulocyte transfusions may be indicated for patients with severe neutropenia, defined as an absolute neutrophil count of $<0.5 \times 10^9$/L, due to congenital or acquired bone marrow failure syndromes with proven or highly probable fungal or bacterial infection is unresponsive to appropriate antimicrobial therapy. Although therapeutic indications for infection form a major group of indications, some centres consider their use in patients for secondary prophylaxis.

Abnormal neutrophil function and persistent infection

Granulocyte transfusions may also be used to support patients with a known congenital disorder of neutrophil function (e.g. chronic granulomatous disease) with infections unresponsive to antimicrobial therapy regardless of their neutrophil count.

Administration of granulocyte concentrates

ABO and RhD-specific granulocyte concentrates (Figure 5.4) should be used following red cell compatibility testing against the patient's serum (because of the high red cell content of the product). Granulocytes should be transfused over 1–2 hours through a standard red cell giving set.

An adequate effective dose is generally considered to be a minimum of 1×10^{10} granulocytes/m^2 body surface area, but transfusion of larger numbers of cells results in higher increments in the absence of alloimmunization. Daily doses of buffy coats

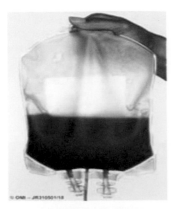

Figure 5.4 Granulocyte concentrate collected by apheresis (courtesy of the Apheresis Team at the Oxford National Blood Service, John Radcliffe Hospital).

(usually 10 donations per dose) may be indicated for larger children (>30 kg) and adults, while unstimulated apheresis donations have sufficient granulocytes to support only small children weighing <30 kg. Stimulated donations from relatives and friends contain considerably higher numbers of granulocytes (see Table 5.2) and may be required only 2–3 times per week. Although, arguably, apheresis collections of granulocytes from stimulated donors are the product of choice for adults, there are major logistic constraints on their collection in the UK. Additionally, G-CSF and corticosteroids are known to cause side effects, and they should be used only in the context of an approved clinical protocol ensuring informed consent and safe donor selection.

Granulocyte transfusions should be discontinued when the neutrophil count recovers, the infection resolves, the patient's condition worsens despite transfusions, or if they provoke severe reactions.

Adverse effects of granulocyte transfusions

Adverse effects of granulocyte transfusions are similar to those caused by platelet transfusions but the reactions are of higher magnitude and severity as they are in part directly proportional to the number of leucocytes present. Furthermore, pulmonary infiltration may result in serious morbidity following granulocyte transfusions.

Pulmonary infiltration results from antibody-mediated sequestration of white cells in the lungs and presents clinically with fluid overload, pulmonary oedema and exacerbation of pre-existing pulmonary pathology. In the most severe form, the adult respiratory distress syndrome may ensue and patients may require ventilatory and/or cardiovascular support.

The development of HLA or HNA alloimmunization in immunosuppressed patients receiving granulocytes transfusion is not a common event. However care should be taken with previously immunized patients since the transfusion of large numbers of leucocytes could trigger a severe and potentially fatal transfusion reaction resembling transfusion-related acute lung injury (see Chapter 11) The high red cell 'contamination' in buffy coat

components may occasionally necessitate venesection, in view of the iatrogenic polycythaemia.

Contraindications to granulocyte transfusions

Transfusion of granulocyte concentrates is not indicated for patients with pyrexia of unknown origin or for sepsis in the absence of neutropenia.

Conclusion

Transfusions of platelet concentrates are life saving in many severely ill patients who are bleeding due to thrombocytopenia. When used to prevent bleeding, platelet transfusions enable the physician to intensify treatment with cytotoxic drugs or the surgeon to operate on a thrombocytopenic patient. Platelet transfusions remain the mainstay of support for thrombocytopenic patients until alternatives currently being developed in the research field – such as growth factor, thrombopoietin or any of the platelet substitutes (lyophilized platelets, infusible platelet membranes, thromboerythrocytes, thrombospheres) – prove to be effective and enter routine clinical practice.

At present, transfusions of granulocyte concentrates are a mode of treatment reserved for desperately ill patients with bacterial or fungal sepsis. Prophylactic granulocyte transfusions cannot currently be recommended due to lack of evidence for benefit.

The correct use of platelets and, in particular, granulocyte concentrates is dependent on careful liaison between experts at regional transfusion centres, hospital transfusion laboratories and clinicians responsible for the care of patients. Inappropriate use of blood components may expose the patient to unnecessary risks and waste scarce resources.

Further reading

British Committee for Standards in Haematology. Guidelines for platelet transfusions. *British Journal of Haematology* 2003; **122**: 10–23.

Dzik S. How I do it: platelet support for refractory patients. *Transfusion* 2007; **47**(3): 374–8.

Price TH. Granulocyte transfusion: current status. *Seminars in Hematology* 2007; **44**: 15–23.

Robinson SP, Marks DI. Granulocyte transfusions in the G-CSF era: where do we stand? *Bone Marrow Transplantation* 2004; **34**(10): 839–46.

Slichter SJ. Platelet transfusion therapy. *Hematology/Oncology Clinics of North America* 2007; **21**(4): 697–729.

Stanworth SJ, Hyde C, Brunskill S, Murphy M. Platelet transfusion prophylaxis for patients with haematological malignancies: where to now? *British Journal of Haematology* 2005; **131**: 588–95.

Stroncek DF, Rebulla P. Platelet transfusions. *Lancet* 2007; **370**(9585): 427–38.

Reference

McClelland DBL (ed.) *Handbook of Transfusion Medicine*, 4th edn. UK Blood Services, London, 2007.

CHAPTER 6

Haemolytic Disease of the Newborn and its Prevention

Fiona Regan, Sailesh Kumar and Marcela Contreras

OVERVIEW

- The most significant cause of haemolytic disease of the fetus and newborn (HDN) is anti-D, caused by maternal alloimmunization to the RhD antigen.
- The introduction of antenatal prophylaxis with anti-D immunoglobulin has been a success story, decreasing the rate of maternal alloimmunization and HDN considerably.
- Routine antenatal prophylaxis, starting at 28 weeks, for all unimmunized D-negative women should prevent alloimmunization even further.
- Antenatal care with strict follow-up of sensitized mothers, as well as fetal medicine units have greatly contributed to the decline in disease severity and mortality.
- Other antibodies that may cause severe HDN are anti-c and anti-K.
- Anti-A and anti-B in group O mothers may lead to HDN, but this is seldom severe.

Aetiology and pathogenesis of haemolytic disease of the newborn

Haemolytic disease of the newborn (HDN) is a condition in which the lifespan of the fetus or infant's red cells is shortened by the action of maternal immunoglobulin G (IgG) red cell alloantibodies, directed against red cell antigens inherited from the father, that cross the placental barrier. The disease begins during intrauterine life. The extent of destruction of fetal red cells varies depending on the specificity, nature and concentration of the maternal antibody. Most maternal red cell antibodies do not cause significant HDN but a few, like anti-D, anti-K and anti-c, may affect the fetus, especially when the antibody concentration is high. In the most severe cases, fetal anaemia and extravascular haemolysis result in hepatosplenomegaly, ascites, subcutaneous oedema, and pleural and pericardial effusions (hydrops fetalis). At present, intrauterine

ABC of Transfusion, 4th edition, 2009. Edited by Marcela Contreras. © 2009 Blackwell Publishing, ISBN: 978-1-4051-5646-2.

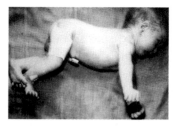

Figure 6.1 Infant with kernicterus (brain damage caused by hyperbilirubinaemia.

death occurs only rarely in developed countries. The clinical picture in less severe cases includes anaemia and postnatal jaundice (due to unconjugated hyperbilirubinaemia not cleared by an immature liver), which, if severe and untreated, can impregnate the basal ganglia, causing spasticity and even kernicterus (Figure 6.1), resulting in death or permanent cerebral damage. In the last 30–40 years, the decline in death rate due to RhD HDN has been substantially greater than the decline in disease.

Although ABO HDN is relatively common, in the UK it is usually mild, affecting the infant, but not the fetus. Many red cell antibody specificities have been reported to cause HDN, but those that most frequently cause significant HDN in people of European origin are anti-D, followed by anti-c and anti-K. The principles of management of HDN are similar regardless of the type of antibody involved, although the disease due to anti-K results in anaemia due to lack of mature red cells, rather than increased red cell destruction as the predominant clinical feature. Anti-K destroys red cell precursors, whereas Rh antibodies destroy mature red cells.

During pregnancy small volumes of fetal red cells pass into the maternal circulation. This transplacental 'leakage' increases as gestation progresses. In the majority of RhD-negative women, an RhD-positive pregnancy does not stimulate the maternal immune system because the volume of red cells that crosses the placenta during pregnancy and at delivery is too low to be immunogenic, either because fetal red cells are rapidly cleared by the maternal mononuclear–phagocytic system or because the woman is a poor responder. Not all RhD-negative mothers are equally at risk of developing anti-D; when the mother is group O and the RhD-positive infant is group A or B, the mother's chances of making anti-D are reduced by a factor of 8 because the maternal anti-AB destroys the fetal red cells that may cross the placenta. In the absence of

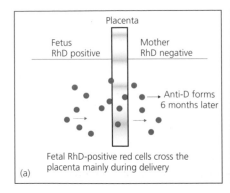

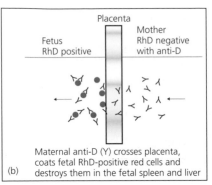

Figure 6.2 Mechanism of (a) RhD sensitization during the first pregnancy and (b) fetal red cell destruction during the second pregnancy with an RhD-positive fetus.

Table 6.1 RhD prophylaxis with anti-D immunoglobulin.

Indication	Dose of anti-D Ig (i.m.)	Comments
Routine antenatal prophylaxis: at 28 and 34 weeks single dose at 28 weeks	500 or 1250 IU preparations ≥1500 IU	28 week dose to be given *after* blood sample for group and antibody screen is taken
Post-delivery	500 IU (covers 4 ml fetal red cells) *or* 1250 IU (covers 10 ml fetal red cells) *or* 1500 IU (covers 12 ml fetal red cells)	Give within 72 hours of delivery, unless the baby is known to be D negative Plus Kleihauer test: additional anti-D needed if fetal bleed is greater than the volume of fetal red cells covered by dose given
Antenatal sensitizing events: before 20 weeks after 20 weeks	250 IU 500, 1250 or 1500 IU	No Kleihauer test or follow-up required Kleihauer test needed: additional anti-D needed if fetal bleed is greater than the volume of fetal red cells covered by dose given Anti-D should be given within 72 hours of the sensitizing event, whatever the gestation

anti-RhD prophylaxis, about 17% of RhD-negative women delivering an ABO-compatible RhD-positive child will have been immunized by the time of a second pregnancy with an RhD-positive child (Figure 6.2). If the child is ABO incompatible, the maternal immunization rate will be much lower. Maternal IgG-1 and -3 anti-D can cross the placenta, enter the fetal circulation and destroy circulating RhD-positive fetal red cells.

Approximately 16% of British white Caucasians are D negative. The D antigen is an integral membrane protein exclusively expressed on red cells and is very immunogenic. In people of European origin, anti-D is by far the commonest cause of HDN.

Immunoprophylaxis

Before immunoprophylaxis became available, the frequency of HDN in the UK was 1% of all births. RhD HDN led to 1.2 deaths per 1000 births in England and Wales. It was shown in the 1960s that sensitization to the D antigen can be prevented by the administration of anti-D immunoglobulin (Ig). When sufficient anti-D Ig is administered to the mother, either intramuscularly or intravenously, within 72 hours of a sensitizing event, immunization can be prevented. Hence, prophylaxis following sensitizing events during pregnancy and postnatal administration of anti-D Ig have

decreased D alloimmunization significantly. Consequently, the incidence of HDN and deaths due to the disease have substantially reduced. The mechanism of prevention of RhD immunization is not clear. Apparently, the anti-D Ig coats the fetal D-positive red cells, which are then rapidly removed from the maternal circulation, before being recognized by the mother's immune system.

Despite a significant reduction in RhD sensitization and HDN with the introduction of postnatal prophylaxis in the early 1970s, a remnant of 1–1.5% of RhD-negative women delivering a second RhD-positive infant became immunized. The most important cause of residual RhD alloimmunization is transplacental leakage of red cells (fetomaternal haemorrhage) during the third trimester, where there has been no overt sensitizing event. It is known that fetomaternal haemorrhages increase as pregnancy advances. Routine antenatal prophylaxis can prevent the vast majority of sensitizations due to fetomaternal red cell leakage in the third trimester.

The current recommendations for anti-D immunoprophylaxis of the Royal College of Obstetricians and Gynaecologists (2002) and the National Institute of Clinical Excellence (2002) are as follows (Table 6.1):

1 Anti-D prophylaxis is recommended for unimmunized D-negative women following the delivery of a D-positive infant,

irrespective of the dose or timing of anti-D Ig administered during pregnancy. A standard dose of at least 500 IU anti-D Ig i.m./i.v. is recommended, followed by a postnatal screening test (usually a Kleihauer test), to identify women who suffer a large fetomaternal haemorrhage and therefore need additional anti-D Ig.

2 Anti-D immunoglobulin is recommended following potentially sensitizing events during pregnancy (Box 6.1).

3 Anti-D prophylaxis is not required for women with threatened miscarriage with a viable fetus and cessation of bleeding during the first trimester.

4 Anti-D prophylaxis is not required following spontaneous complete miscarriages during the first trimester if there is no clinical intervention to aid or complete uterine evacuation.

5 Routine antenatal anti-D prophylaxis (RAADP) is recommended for all non-sensitized D-negative women. The protocol depends on the dose used: (i) one dose of 1500 IU i.m. or i.v. anti-D Ig at 28 weeks' gestation; or (ii) two doses of <1500 IU i.m. or i.v. anti-D Ig, one at 28 and the other at 34 weeks' gestation.

Sensitizing events include threatened miscarriage continuing into the second trimester, spontaneous miscarriages after the first trimester, assisted evacuation of the uterus at any time in pregnancy, abortions at any time of gestation, ectopic pregnancy, invasive prenatal procedures (chorionic villus sampling, amniocentesis, etc.), antepartum haemorrhage, external cephalic version, closed abdominal injury and intrauterine injury.

Preparation, dose and administration of anti-D Ig to RhD-negative women

Anti-D Ig is manufactured from plasma collected from non-UK donors who have been hyperimmunized to attain high levels of anti-D. There are four virally inactivated polyclonal anti-D Ig preparations licensed for use in the UK. Anti-D Ig is normally given intramuscularly and 125 IU can suppress immunization by 1 ml of D-positive red cells, if given within 72 hours of a sensitizing event.

Most fetomaternal haemorrhages (FMH) involve <4 ml of fetal red cells, so a dose of 500 IU anti-D Ig will prevent most maternal immunizations.

Large fetomaternal bleeds at delivery

A cord blood sample should be tested at delivery to identify all D-positive infants so that their mothers can be given a dose of at least 500 IU of anti-D Ig. This is sufficient for 99.4% of women who have an FMH of less than 4 ml. To ensure that the remaining 0.6% of women are identified, all D-negative women delivering a D-positive infant must have a blood sample taken within 1–2 hours of delivery to establish the volume of FMH. Frequently, the acid elution test of Kleihauer, which detects fetal red cells (Figure 6.3), is used. Flow cytometry, which detects D-positive red cells (Figure 6.4), is also appropriate though more complex and expensive for routine use. If the Kleihauer test suggests

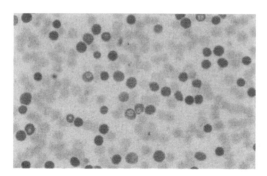

Figure 6.3 Kleihauer staining to show fetal red cells (dark staining) among maternal red cells (pale 'ghosts').

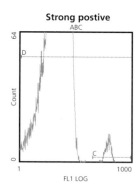

750 counts in RhD +ve zone (total 60,000)
= 125% ≡ 27ml FMH

Figure 6.4 Flow cytometry detects D-positive red cells.

Box 6.1 **Indications for administering anti-D Ig to unimmunized D-negative women**

- Delivery of a D-positive baby: a standard dose of at least 500 IU anti-D Ig
- Routine antenatal prophylaxis at 28 and 34 weeks' gestation if the dose used is <1500 IU. A single dose at 28 weeks is sufficient if the dose is ≥1500 IU.
- Potentially sensitizing events during pregnancy:
  - therapeutic termination of pregnancy (surgical or medical methods)
  - ectopic pregnancy
  - spontaneous miscarriage after 12 weeks' gestation
  - spontaneous miscarriage before 12 weeks' gestation if evacuation is assisted by surgical or medical intervention
  - threatened miscarriage after 12 weeks' gestation
  - threatened miscarriage before 12 weeks' gestation if bleeding is heavy or associated with abdominal pain, especially if nearing 12 weeks' gestation
  - invasive prenatal diagnostic procedures (chorionic villus sampling, amniocentesis, fetal blood sampling)
  - other intrauterine procedures (insertion of shunts, embryo reduction)
  - antepartum haemorrhage
  - external cephalic version of the fetus
  - closed abdominal injury
  - intrauterine death or stillbirth.

a bleed of >4 ml, the volume of the FMH should be confirmed by flow cytometry. National External Quality Assurance Scheme (NEQAS) results suggest that flow cytometry assessments may be more reliable for large FMHs (>4 ml), but not as good for small volume ones. However, flow cytometry is useful for FMH quantitation where the mother has hereditary persistence of fetal haemoglobin resulting in a false high Kleihauer result. The test for quantitation of FMH must be done promptly enough to allow sufficient time to give any additional anti-D Ig required, within 72 hours of delivery. Note that 0.3% of women have an FMH of >15 ml, so even when an intramuscular preparation containing 1500 IU anti-D Ig is used a test to quantitate the size of the FMH must still be performed.

For very large FMHs, sufficient anti-D Ig can either be given intramuscularly using higher dose preparations in a small volume, e.g. a 2500 IU i.m.; or an intravenous anti-D Ig may be given. There are two advantages of using i.v. anti-D Ig for large FMHs:

1 As the full dose of anti-D reaches the circulation immediately, only half the intramuscular dose is required. Following an intramuscular injection, absorption of anti-D Ig is both slower and may be incomplete.
2 Large doses of anti-D Ig can be given without resorting to multiple, painful intramuscular injections.

When additional anti-D Ig is given, a repeat Kleihauer test should be done to establish clearance of all D-positive red cells from the maternal circulation. A Kleihauer test is recommended 72 hours after the additional dose if anti-D Ig is given intramuscularly, or 48 hours later if anti-D Ig is given intravascularly. If the Kleihauer test shows fetal red cells, the volume of residual D-positive red cells should be determined by flow cytometry and further anti-D Ig given, as required.

Sensitizing events after 20 weeks' gestation

If sensitizing events during a pregnancy that take place after 20 weeks' gestation, a dose of at least 500 IU anti-D Ig i.m. should be given; a Kleihauer test is also required. Anti-D Ig should be given within 72 hours of the sensitizing event.

Sensitizing events before 20 weeks' gestation

If sensitizing events during pregnancy, if occurring before 20 weeks' gestation, no Kleihauer test is required as the fetal blood volume is small. A dose of 250 IU anti-D is sufficient for prophylaxis.

Other red cell alloantibodies causing HDN

Most IgG red cell alloantibodies have been reported to cause HDN. However, the non-D alloantibodies commonly implicated in causing haemolytic disease of the fetus and newborn include anti-K, anti-c, anti-E and ABO isoantibodies. HDN due to most alloantibodies is characterized by anaemia and hyperbilirubinaemia in the newborn infant. However, in HDN due to Kell antibodies (anti-K, -k, -Kp^a, -Kp^b, etc.), anaemia is the predominant feature and a few cases of *hydrops fetalis* have been reported. Kell antibodies have a predilection for red cell progenitors, causing significant suppression of erythropoiesis and relatively modest peripheral

haemolysis. Most Kell antibodies are stimulated by a previous transfusion. Hence, once anti-Kell is detected in maternal blood the partner's phenotype should be tested, and if his red cells test positive for the corresponding antigen referral to a specialist fetal medicine unit is advisable. Although the risk of significant haemolysis is low at indirect antiglobulin titres of less than 32, it is good practice to follow up the trend of the antibody level and start non-invasive monitoring of the fetus for signs of anaemia. Ultrasonography and non-invasive middle cerebral artery Doppler velocimetry are used to monitor the development of fetal anaemia (see Chapter 7). With c alloimmunization the risk of fetal anaemia is somewhat higher when the anti-c level exceeds 7.5 IU/ml, and fetal monitoring is recommended.

ABO haemolytic disease of the newborn

In the UK one in three fetuses are ABO incompatible with their mother, but ABO HDN is uncommon because most maternal anti-A and anti-B is IgM and cannot cross the placenta. Moreover, A and B antigens are distributed in tissue and body fluids, thus competing for antibodies that may cross the placenta. Also, A and B antigens are poorly expressed on fetal red cells. However, some group O women (particularly of Asian and African origin) have high levels of anti-A and anti-B, with a significant IgG component. This may result in ABO HDN. Unlike the situation with other alloantibodies, ABO HDN may occur in the first or subsequent pregnancies, but is rarely severe and has not been reported to damage the fetus significantly. Maternal ABO antibody level does not correlate with fetal/neonatal anaemia and testing the level of maternal ABO antibodies during pregnancy is not recommended. However, if an infant develops unexplained clinical jaundice within a few days of delivery, ABO HDN should be considered. The mother is always group O and the baby is group A or B. Often, the direct antiglobulin test (DAT) on the baby's red cells is negative, but a moderate or weakly positive DAT is seen in moderate or severe HDN. Spherocytosis in the infant's blood film is characteristic of ABO HDN (Figure 6.5). Phototherapy may be required (Figure 6.6), but exchange transfusion is rarely needed (see Chapter 7).

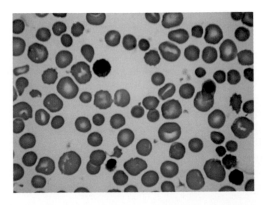

Figure 6.5 Blood film showing spherocytosis in ABO haemolytic disease of the newborn.

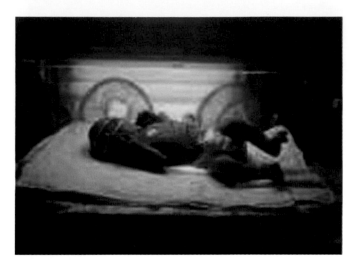

Figure 6.6 A jaundiced infant receiving phototherapy.

Blood grouping and antibody screening in pregnancy

At the first visit (usually 12–16 weeks) all pregnant women should have blood taken for ABO and D blood grouping and red cell antibody screening, in addition to other antenatal tests. Approximately 97% of women will have no detectable red cell alloantibodies at booking. Subsequent monitoring is indicated in Figure 6.7. If anti-D or anti-c are found at booking, their levels should be quantitated and the antibody trend followed up throughout pregnancy. D-negative women with no anti-D at booking are candidates for routine antenatal RhD prophylaxis at 28 weeks. It is now possible to know the RhD type of the fetus by non-invasive, sensitive molecular typing of fetal DNA in maternal plasma; if the fetus is RhD negative, antenatal prophylaxis is not needed. There should be close collaboration between the obstetric unit and the blood transfusion department, preferably with named individuals responsible for following up abnormal results and identifying women eligible for anti-D prophylaxis. This is particularly important as many women,

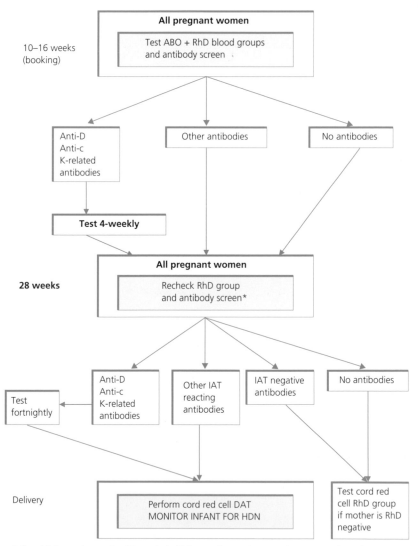

Figure 6.7 Action chart for blood grouping and antibody testing during pregnancy. Since most anti-K antibodies are stimulated by a previous transfusion, if the partner is proven to be K negative and there is certainty that he is the father of the child, regular antibody monitoring can be abandoned. DAT, direct antiglobulin test; IAT, indirect antiglobulin test.

* If anti-D is not detected at 28 weeks in RhD-negative mothers, routine antenatal prophylaxis should commence.

Box 6.2 **Post-delivery cord blood tests to be undertaken if the mother has clinically significant antibody/ies**

- Direct antiglobulin test or DAT (positive if baby has corresponding antigen/s).
- If the DAT is positive, test:
  - haemoglobulin
  - bilirubin
  - blood film (spherocytes are present if there is significant haemolysis)

particularly those from immigrant or travelling communities, may either book late or have very fragmented antenatal care, and may fall through the system unless special safeguards are in place. Every Trust with an obstetric department should have a named obstetrician/fetal medicine specialist as well as a haematologist or transfusion medicine consultant from whom advice can be obtained about HDN. Previous obstetric history (severe fetal or neonatal anaemia, severe jaundice, etc.) is also particularly important and the relevant patients should be identified early in the pregnancy so that appropriate serological and fetal monitoring can be instituted. When a pregnant woman is found to have atypical antibodies, the laboratory report should state the specificity and clinical significance of these antibodies.

Post-delivery tests

Infants born to women who have clinically significant antibodies should have a cord blood sample taken for a DAT (Box 6.2). If the DAT is negative, HDN is unlikely. A positive DAT is not diagnostic of HDN; it only signifies the coating of the infant's red cells with maternally derived antibody. When the DAT is positive, the infant's haemoglobin and bilirubin levels should be tested to diagnose HDN. Examining a blood film is useful in diagnosing ABO HDN. The treatment of mild to moderate HDN is phototherapy. Exchange transfusion is indicated for severe HDN and top-up transfusions are indicated if anaemia persists in the infant (see Chapter 7).

The future

The very significant reduction in the incidence and deaths due to HDN over the past 30–40 years is a result of both anti-D immunoprophylaxis and improved antenatal care and management of sick fetuses and infants. In the near future sensitive molecular techniques on maternal plasma will allow routine determination of the D type of fetuses carried by D-negative mothers, thus avoiding antenatal prophylaxis when the fetus is D negative. Unfortunately, monoclonal anti-D for prophylaxis does not seem to be in the horizon. In recent years the labelling of all blood bags in England and Wales with the full Rh and K type has meant that K-negative women of childbearing potential can be given K-negative blood, which should further reduce the burden of HDN.

Further reading

British Committee for Standards in Haematology, Blood Transfusion Task Force. Guidelines for blood grouping and red cell antibody testing during pregnancy. *Transfusion Medicine* 1996; **6**: 71–4.

Clarke CA. Preventing rhesus babies: the Liverpool research and follow up. *Archives of Disease in Childhood* 1989; **64**: 1734–40.

Joint working group of the British Blood Transfusion Society and the Royal College of Obstetricians and Gynaecologists. Recommendations for the use of anti-D immunoglobulin for Rh prophylaxis. *Transfusion Medicine* 1999: **9**; 93–7.

Mollison PL, Engelfriet CP, Contreras M. *Blood Transfusion in Clinical Medicine,* 10th edn. Blackwell Science, Oxford, 1997.

National Institute of Clinical Excellence (NICE). *Pregnancy: Routine anti-D prophylaxis for rhesus negative women.* NICE Guidelines No. 41. NICE Publications, London, 2002.

Royal College of Obstetricians and Gynaecologists (RCOG) *Anti-D Immunoglobulin for Rh Prophylaxis.* RCOG Green Top Guidelines. RCOG Publications, London, 2002.

Vaughan JI, Warwich R, Letsky EA, Nicolini U, Rodeck CH, Fiasco NM. Erythropoiesis suppression in foetal anaemia because of Kell alloimmunisation. *Journal of Obstetrics and Gynaecology* 1994; **171**: 247–52.

CHAPTER 7

Fetal and Neonatal Transfusion

Helen V. New and Sailesh Kumar

OVERVIEW

- Fetuses and neonates are amongst the most vulnerable transfusion recipients.

- Special blood components are available in order to minimize the risks of transfusion. It is important to increase awareness of these in order to ensure selection of the appropriate component.

- Fetal transfusions are highly specialized procedures, with a risk of fetal loss of at least 1% from each procedure.

- Fetuses may be transfused with either red cells or platelets. Red cell intrauterine transfusions have decreased following the introduction of routine anti-D for all RhD-negative women. Monitoring for fetal anaemia is now by non-invasive Doppler ultrasound of blood flow in the middle cerebral artery.

- Sick babies in neonatal units are frequently transfused but guidelines on transfusion indications are still largely based on consensus and expert opinion.

- Strategies to reduce neonatal transfusion include local guidelines to minimize the frequency and volume of blood taken for testing.

Fetal transfusions are highly specialized procedures, performed in only a few fetal medicine centres in the UK. On the other hand, infants in neonatal units are frequently transfused, so optimizing neonatal transfusions is an issue for many hospitals. Fetuses and neonates are among the most vulnerable recipients of the infectious, metabolic or immunological complications of blood transfusion. Moreover, problems with long-term side effects, including some infections, are likely to be greatest for this population as most will live for several decades after transfusion.

Special components are required for fetuses and neonates in order to minimize the risks of transfusion (see Table 7.1 for discussion), and these are described in detail in the 2004 British Committee for Standards in Haematology (BCSH) guidelines on transfusion for neonates and older children.

Fetal transfusion

Intrauterine transfusions may use either red cells to correct fetal anaemia such as caused by maternal red cell alloantibodies causing haemolytic disease or, more rarely, platelets when there is fetal alloimmune thrombocytopenia. Routine antenatal and postnatal anti-D immunoglobulin (Ig) prophylaxis for all Rh-negative women (see Chapter 6) has decreased the incidence of haemolytic disease of the fetus and newborn, so the number of red cell intrauterine transfusions has decreased markedly over the last 20 years.

Red cell transfusion

The commonest cause of fetal anaemia is haemolytic disease caused by red cell alloantibodies, although it may also occur following fetal infection with parvovirus B19, or be due to congenital red cell aplasia. Survival rates of fetuses with anaemia have improved considerably since the introduction of intrauterine transfusion. Pregnancies complicated by red cell alloantibodies (particularly anti-D, anti-c and anti-K) may result in fetal anaemia secondary to transplacental passage of maternal IgG antibodies that bind to red cells carrying paternal antigens, leading to progressive fetal haemolysis. In severe cases the anaemic fetus develops ascites, subcutaneous oedema, and pleural and pericardial effusions (hydrops fetalis), and may die *in utero* (see Chapter 6).

The main advance in the management of pregnancies at risk of anaemia or where anaemia is suspected is the use of weekly fetal middle cerebral artery monitoring (Figure 7.1). Middle cerebral artery peak systolic velocities (Doppler) are raised in anaemic fetuses, and values greater than 1.5 MoM (multiples of the median) for the specific gestation are predictive of moderate or severe fetal anaemia with 100% sensitivity and a false positive rate of 12%. Middle cerebral artery Doppler results show very good correlation with amniotic fluid bilirubin levels. This non-invasive method has supplanted the traditional technique of serial amniocentesis for bilirubin measurement.

Fetal blood sampling and intrauterine transfusion

If middle cerebral artery monitoring suggests anaemia, fetal blood sampling and intrauterine transfusion are indicated. The risks of the procedure depend on the age of gestation, the site of sampling and underlying pathology. The risk of fetal loss from uncomplicated fetal blood sampling is between 1% and 3%; however if the

ABC of Transfusion, 4th edition, 2009. Edited by Marcela Contreras. © 2009 Blackwell Publishing, ISBN: 978-1-4051-5646-2.

Table 7.1 Some of the requirements to consider for fetal and neonatal blood components.

Issue to consider	Component specification
Blood group compatibility	Use red cells compatible with any maternal antibodies, e.g. anti-A, anti-B, anti-D or anti-c (usually give group O RhD negative in the absence of significant maternal antibodies)
Reduction of risk of morbidity from antibodies in donor plasma	Screen donors for high titre anti-A, anti-B and atypical antibodies. For neonates who are not group O, do not use group O FFP and avoid group O platelets where possible
Reduction of infection risk	Leucodepleted; CMV negative; 'accredited' donors who have donated at least twice in the previous 2 years; methylene blue-treated FFP imported from the USA
Age of red cells	Use fresh blood (<5 days old) for fetal and large volume neonatal transfusions. Extracellular potassium levels rise during red cell storage. Red cells for top-up transfusion can be of any age, since it is better to dedicate paedipaks from the same donor for one recipient (Figure 7.3)
Suspension medium for red cells	Use citrate-phosphate-dextrose (CPD) for IUT and neonatal exchange transfusions; saline-adenine-glucose-mannitol (SAG-M) for neonatal top-up transfusions (see text)
Haematocrit of packed red cells	High (0.70–0.85) for IUT, to reduce volume overload Intermediate (0.5–0.6) for neonatal exchange transfusion Broader range (0.5–0.7) for neonatal top-up transfusion
Prevention of transfusion-associated graft-versus-host disease	Irradiate red cells and platelets for IUT, any neonatal transfusion post IUT, exchange transfusions and some immunodeficiency states

CMV, cytomegalovirus; FFP, fresh frozen plasma; IUT, intrauterine transfusion.

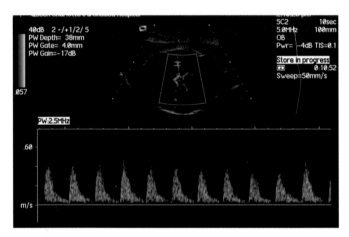

Figure 7.1 Circle of Willis in the fetus with the cursor placed on the middle cerebral artery, and the Doppler waveform.

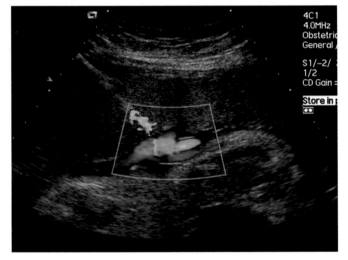

Figure 7.2 Fetal blood sampling from the placental cord insertion site.

fetus is hydropic the risk may be as high as 20%. These are difficult procedures and should be performed by fetal medicine specialists in selected tertiary centres. Transfusions are started as late in pregnancy as possible (ideally after at least 18 weeks' gestation), and the intervals between transfusions should be maximized by giving as many red cells as possible in the allowed volume, i.e. using packed cells with a high haematocrit (0.70–0.85%).

Sampling can be performed from either the placental cord insertion site (Figure 7.2) or the intrahepatic vein. The intrahepatic approach is less likely to cause fetal complications but is technically more challenging. Complications of fetal blood sampling include fetal bradycardia, haemorrhage, cord haematoma, cardiac tamponade and fetal death. There may also be increased maternal alloimmunization. The procedure is done under continuous ultrasound guidance and facilities for immediate analysis of the fetal blood should be available.

Irradiated, group O blood, negative for cytomegalovirus (CMV), which should be less than 5 days old and which has been crossmatched with a maternal plasma sample, is used for fetal transfusion. A final post-transfusion fetal haematocrit of around 0.45% is desirable. Transfusions may be given intravascularly (for immediate correction) or may be combined with concomitant intraperitoneal administration (when blood is slowly absorbed through the lymphatics). This combination increases the interval between transfusions by maintaining adequate haemoglobin concentrations for longer. Although the timing of subsequent transfusions is dependent on the rate of decline of the fetal haematocrit, the presence of hydrops, and gestational age, in general a 3–5-weekly interval is the norm. Close monitoring with middle cerebral artery Doppler is essential and allows precise timing of further intervention.

Overall, fetal hydrops usually reverses after one or two transfusions, and survival is about 85%, with a survival rate of greater than 90% when there has been severe disease but no hydrops.

Platelet transfusion

Fetal platelet transfusions are used for fetomaternal alloimmune thrombocytopenia. This is a rare condition due to maternal alloimmunization to fetal platelet antigens inherited from the father, and occurs in approximately one in 1000 to one in 1500 live births. The most common human platelet antigens involved are HPA-1a (85% of cases) and HPA-5b (10% of cases). Affected fetuses have a 10–30% risk of intracranial haemorrhage either antenatally or peripartum. There is uncertainty over the optimal antenatal management, which may include maternal treatment with intravenous Ig, with or without steroids, and intrauterine platelet transfusions. Many centres start with intravenous Ig, and if there is a poor response of the fetal platelet count will then add in steroids or move to weekly platelet transfusions until delivery.

The risks of intrauterine platelet transfusions in this case are similar to those of red cell transfusion, with a risk of fetal loss of at least 1% from each procedure. The platelets used are group-appropriate, negative for the platelet antigen to which the mother has made antibody, CMV negative, irradiated and concentrated.

Neonatal transfusion

Sick neonates are frequently transfused, but guidelines on transfusion indications (such as from the BCSH, 2004) are still largely based on consensus and expert opinion. There is evidence from reports to the UK Serious Hazards of Transfusion (SHOT) haemovigilance scheme that there are a disproportionately high number of transfusion errors in this age group, mostly due to transfusion of the wrong blood component. It is therefore important to increase awareness of the components available and to ensure that such transfusions are only given in situations that are accepted as appropriate.

Red cell transfusions

Because of concerns in the UK regarding possible transfusion transmission of variant Creutzfeldt–Jakob disease (vCJD) all blood is leucodepleted. Further measures are being taken to reduce the exposure of children to UK plasma as apparently most residual infectivity is present in plasma. The use of packed red cells in additive solution (saline adenine glucose mannitol or SAG-M), which contains very little residual plasma, is being encouraged where possible, rather than the use of red cells in anticoagulant (citrate phosphate dextrose or CPD), which may have significantly more plasma. Although there have been concerns over possible toxicity to neonates of the SAG-M constituents, they have been shown to be safe for small volume neonatal top-up transfusions. There is also evidence that they are safe for large volume transfusions in neonatal cardiac surgery (Mou et al. 2004), and the use of red cells in SAG-M is now recommended by the BCSH for this indication. However, for fetal transfusions and neonatal exchange transfusions red cells in CPD are still recommended, as the effect of additives in these situations is more uncertain.

Table 7.2 Suggested transfusion thresholds for neonates.

	Transfusion threshold
Transfusion of red blood cells	
Anaemia in the first 24 hours	Hb < 12 g/dl
Neonate receiving mechanical ventilation	Hb < 12 g/dl
Acute blood loss	≥10% blood volume lost
Oxygen dependency (not ventilated)	Hb < 8–11 g/dl (depending on clinical situation)
Late anaemia, stable patient (off oxygen)	Hb < 7 g/dl
Transfusion of platelets	
Consider in all neonates	<30 platelets × 10^9/L
Consider if increased bleeding risk, for example:	<50 platelets × 10^9/L
• <1000 g and <1 week of age	
• clinically unstable (e.g. labile blood pressure)	
• previous major bleeding (e.g. grade 3–4 intraventricular haemorrhage)	
• current minor bleeding (e.g. petechiae)	
• coagulopathy	
• planned surgery or exchange transfusion	
Major bleeding	<100 platelets × 10^9/L

Adapted from BCSH (2004) and Murray and Roberts (2004).
There is little clear evidence for much of this guidance, particularly regarding long-term outcomes, but they may serve as a starting point for developing local guidelines.

Small volume top-ups

Most red cell transfusions to neonates are small volume top-ups (10–20 ml/kg) for preterm babies. These transfusions are frequently given to treat anaemia from repeated blood sampling, but may also be required for other causes of anaemia such as prematurity, haemolysis, congenital infections or genetic disorders. The triggers for transfusion in these babies vary, depending on factors such as the age of the baby and the cardiorespiratory status (Table 7.2). They are mostly based on observational clinical studies and vary between units, with a general trend towards a more restrictive use of red cells over recent years.

Strict adherence to transfusion guidelines has been shown to reduce the number of transfusions given to neonates, and this should be coupled with local strategies to minimize the frequency and volume of blood taken for testing. The use of paedipaks (Figure 7.3) reduces donor exposure as multiple transfusions from one donor can be given to the same neonate over a period of several weeks.

Large volume transfusions

Neonates are given large volume transfusions (may be as much as two blood volumes) in the settings of exchange transfusion, cardiac surgery and sometimes during resuscitation or other surgery (Figure 7.4). They should have blood of neonatal specification, which also needs to be fresh (less than 5 days old) in order not to have problems due to high potassium (see Table 7.1). When phototherapy fails, exchange transfusions are undertaken to treat hyperbilirubinaemia, with or without anaemia, for example in

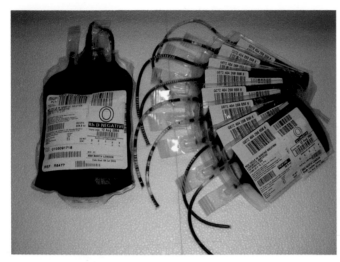

Figure 7.3 A set of eight paedipaks split from a single unit of red cells. (Courtesy of Jan Green, National Blood Service.)

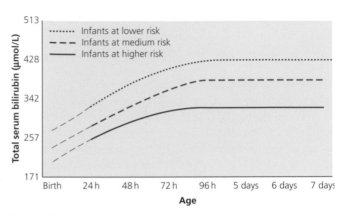

Figure 7.5 Example guideline for exchange transfusion, taking into account the level of bilirubin and the age of the infant. This graph is for infants of 35 weeks' gestation or more. The dashed lines for the first 24 hours indicate uncertainty due to a wide range of clinical circumstances and a range of responses to phototherapy. (Adapted from American Academy of Pediatrics 2004.)

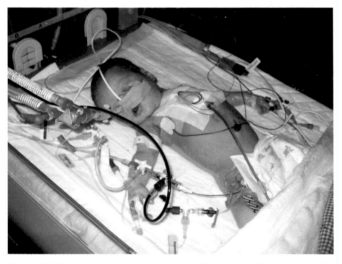

Figure 7.4 Transfusion of a neonate post cardiac surgery. (Courtesy of Ruth Allis.)

haemolytic disease of the newborn (HDN). The indication for exchange transfusion for hyperbilirubinaemia will depend on the bilirubin level and the gestation and age of the baby; there are charts and guidelines for neonatologists to follow in this situation (see, for example, Figure 7.5). General experience in undertaking this procedure is decreasing and it is important to establish local practice guidelines.

The optimum haematocrit of the red cells used for exchange will vary depending on the level of anaemia of the neonate. The exchange procedure can be modified as appropriate by including saline if the haematocrit is too high for a given situation. Therefore it is important for the blood provided to have a tightly controlled haematocrit in order to provide accurate information for neonatologists. The BCSH guidelines currently recommend 0.5–0.6, and the National Blood Service (NBS) has to narrow this range still further, to 0.50–0.55.

Platelets

Platelets are given to a significant number of neonates on neonatal units, largely for prophylaxis in the absence of bleeding, with transfusion rates of up to 9% reported in neonatal intensive care units. The common indications vary depending on whether the baby is term or preterm, but include thrombocytopenia due to perinatal asphyxia and sepsis. It is particularly important to remember fetomaternal alloimmune thrombocytopenia (known as neonatal alloimmune thrombocytopenia, or NAITP), which is usually detected in otherwise well term babies, as transfusions with platelets negative for the common human platelet antigens involved (HPA-1a and HPA-5b) are indicated and are specially provided by the NBS for this situation.

The platelet count at which it is appropriate to transfuse neonates is unclear. The few data from randomized studies suggest that there is no benefit in transfusing preterm babies with platelet counts greater than 50×10^9/L in order to reduce intracranial haemorrhage. Below this level, guidelines such as those from the BCSH recommend a threshold of $20–30 \times 10^9$/L, depending on the clinical situation (see Table 7.2). An observational study has recently been undertaken in the UK to look at the indications and outcome for neonatal platelet transfusions; it may be possible to use this as the basis for future randomized studies in this area.

Platelets for neonates follow the neonatal criteria as in Table 7.1, and are quarter splits of a single apheresis donation. Babies who are deemed likely to have several transfusions over a short time should be given more than one transfusion from the same donor, where possible.

Fresh frozen plasma

Accepted indications for the use of fresh frozen plasma (FFP) on neonatal units have become more restricted over recent years, such that it is no longer considered appropriate to use it as a volume expander or during partial exchange transfusions for polycythaemia. Current guidelines recommend FFP primarily for bleeding as a result of vitamin K deficiency and for bleeding or

Table 7.3 Comparison of neonatal and adult laboratory coagulation ranges.

(a) Figures for adults and healthy full-term infants during the first month of life.

Test	Postnatal age			Adult
	Day 1	Day 5	Day 30	
PT (s)	13.0 (10.1–15.9)	12.4 (10.0–15.3)	11.8 (10.0–14.3)	12.4 (10.8–13.9)
APTT (s)	42.9 (31.3–54.5)	42.6 (25.4–59.8)	40.4 (32.0–55.2)	33.5 (26.6–40.3)
Fibrinogen (g/L)	2.83 (1.67–3.99)	3.12 (1.62–4.62)	2.70 (1.62–3.78)	2.78 (1.56–4.00)

(b) Figures for healthy preterm infants (30–36 weeks gestation) during the first month of life.

Test	Postnatal age		
	Day 1	Day 5	Day 30
PT (s)	13.0 (10.6–16.2)	12.5 (10.0–15.3)	11.8 (10.0–13.6)
APTT (s)	53.6 (27.5–79.4)	50.5 (26.9–74.1)	44.7 (26.9–62.5)
Fibrinogen (g/L)	2.43 (1.50–3.73)	2.80 (1.60–4.18)	2.54 (1.50–4.14)

APTT, activated partial thromboplastin time; PT, prothrombin time.
Data from Andrew et al. (1988, 1990), expressed as means followed by ranges which include 95% of the population. Each mean value is based on tests from a minimum of 40 infants, all of whom received 1 mg vitamin K intramuscularly at birth. The few data available for earlier gestational ages show even more prolonged laboratory coagulation times (Andrew et al. 1990). Coagulation results are technique dependent and will vary between laboratories. However, it is difficult to create local neonatal coagulation ranges, so these ranges are often used to give local comparative guidance.

significant bleeding risk where there are coagulopathies such as disseminated intravascular coagulation. However, it is important to remember that the laboratory coagulation screening times, in particular the activated partial thromboplastin time (APTT), may be significantly longer than in adults, depending on the gestational and postnatal age of the baby (Table 7.3). It is therefore important to interpret coagulation results on these babies with caution, and the use of an APTT ratio based on adult ranges is likely to be particularly misleading when trying to diagnose a coagulopathy in a preterm baby.

There is little evidence from randomized trials regarding the use of FFP for neonates apart from the large prospective study undertaken by the Northern Neonatal Nursing Initiative (NNNI) Trial Group (1996), which showed no benefit from the use of prophylactic FFP given to preterm babies to prevent intraventricular haemorrhage. This study did not include coagulation testing, so a subset of babies with a coagulopathy might have benefited. Overall, the use of FFP for neonates is of uncertain benefit in most situations and its use should be minimized where possible, taking into account neonatal coagulation ranges and the clinical status of the baby.

The component provided by the NBS is methylene blue-treated FFP imported from the USA in order to minimize the risk of transfusion-transmitted infection including vCJD (Figure 7.6). The ABO blood group should be compatible with the baby for FFP and cryoprecipitate.

Cryoprecipitate may be given to neonates with low fibrinogen levels (<1 g/L) and a risk of bleeding. As it is usually given in situations where babies are also receiving FFP, it is desirable to give cryoprecipitate only if the neonatal fibrinogen level remains low despite FFP transfusion.

Prescribing and administration

As discussed above, the indications for neonatal transfusion are not always clear-cut. It is therefore particularly important to record clearly the clinical reasons for transfusion and the clinical and laboratory outcomes. Local guidelines on transfusion indications should be followed, and ways of reducing transfusions such as by reducing blood sampling should be maximized. A common error is the selection of an incorrect blood component for transfusion, so it is important to ensure good training of junior doctors, nurses and laboratory staff. In addition, neonatal components must be prescribed correctly, and both the volume and time taken for the transfusion should be recorded in order to prevent incidents such as adult 'units' being given inappropriately quickly to a small baby (Table 7.4). Communication between neonatal units and blood banks needs to be close in order to make the best use of the allocation and use of red cell paedipaks.

All neonatal blood components should be transfused via a 170–200 μm filter. Ideally this is part of a specific paediatric giving set with small priming volumes (Figure 7.7), but if such sets are not available the blood component can be drawn from the bag through a separate filter into a syringe and then delivered through a syringe driver. If a paediatric giving set is used, blood can be delivered either through a syringe driver or through a suitable volumetric pump (refer to local guidelines).

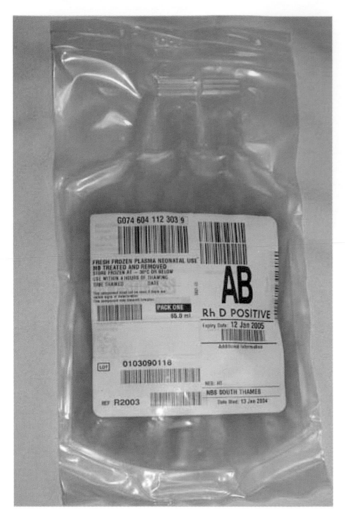

Figure 7.6 Neonatal fresh frozen plasma. (Courtesy of the National Blood Service.)

Table 7.4 Suggested volumes and rates of neonatal transfusions. These give general guidance, and the actual values used will depend on the clinical status of the baby at the time.

Component	Volume usually administered	Rate
Red cell concentrates		
(1) Exchange transfusion	80–100 ml/kg (for anaemia) 160–200 ml/kg (for hyperbilirubinaemia)	Depends on stability of baby: discuss with NICU consultant
(2) Top-up transfusion	10–20 ml/kg*	5 ml/kg/h†
(3) Emergency large volume transfusion	10–20 ml/kg	Rapid infusion only for resuscitation
Platelet concentrates	10–20 ml/kg	10–20 ml/kg/h
Fresh frozen plasma	10–20 ml/kg	10–20 ml/kg/h
Cryoprecipitate	5–10 ml/kg	10–20 ml/kg/h (i.e. over approx 30–60 min)

NICU, neonatal intensive care unit.

*May also use the formula:
Volume of packed cells (ml) = weight (kg) × desired rise in haemoglobin × 4.
†Furosemide is sometimes used, e.g. ventilation with acute respiratory distress.

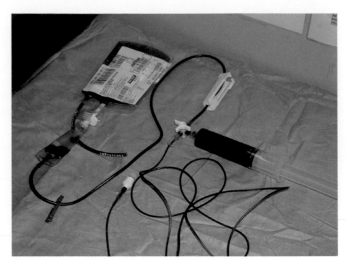

Figure 7.7 Example of an administration set for neonatal transfusion. The red cell paedipak is attached to a paediatric giving set with an integral 200 μm filter and three-way tap. In this case the blood is then drawn into a syringe for administration to the baby using a syringe driver, but the giving set is also suitable for use with an appropriate volumetric pump. (Courtesy of Rachel Moss, St Mary's Hospital.)

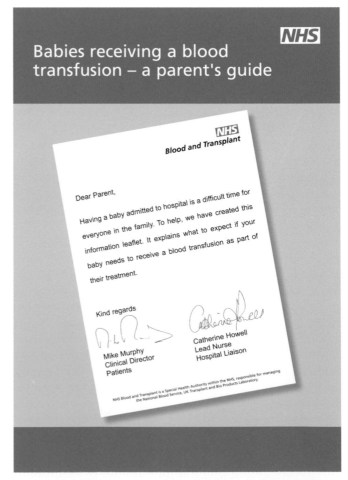

Figure 7.8 Cover of the parent information leaflet on neonatal transfusion provided by the National Blood Service. (Courtesy of the National Blood Service.)

Parents are not generally required to give written consent for transfusion in the UK, but it is very important that the transfusion should be discussed with them in advance. To help with this process, the NBS has produced a parent information sheet to be made available to clinicians in hospitals (Figure 7.8).

Conclusion

Fetal and neonatal transfusions are specialized interventions, with long-term benefits when used appropriately. Despite the fact that only a small proportion of transfusions are given to this patient population they are often relatively complex, and require close attention in order to perform them correctly.

Acknowledgments

We are grateful to Sunit Godambe and Rachel Moss for comments on the text.

Further reading

British Committee for Standards in Haematology (BCSH). Transfusion guidelines for neonates and older children. *British Journal of Haematology* 2004; **124**: 433–53.

Bullock R, Martin WL, Coomarasamy A, Kilby MD. Prediction of fetal anemia in pregnancies with red-cell alloimmunization: comparison of middle cerebral artery peak systolic velocity and amniotic fluid OD450. *Ultrasound in Obstetrics and Gynecology* 2005; **25**: 331–4.

Mari G, Deter RL, Carpenter RL, et al. Noninvasive diagnosis by Doppler ultrasonography of fetal anemia due to maternal red-cell alloimmunization. Collaborative Group for Doppler Assessment of the Blood Velocity in Anemic Fetuses. *New England Journal of Medicine* 2000; **342**: 9–14.

Maxwell DJ, Johnson P, Hurley P, Neales K, Allan L, Knott P. Fetal blood sampling and pregnancy loss in relation to indication. *British Journal of Obstetrics and Gynaecology* 1991; **98**: 892–7.

Murray NA, Roberts IA: Neonatal transfusion practice. *Archives of Disease in Childhood Fetal Neonatal Edition* 2004; **89**: F101–F107.

New HV. Paediatric transfusion. *Vox Sanguinis* 2006; **90**: 1–9.

References

American Academy of Pediatrics. American Academy of Pediatrics guideline: management of hyperbilirubinemia in the newborn infant 35 weeks or more weeks of gestation. *Pediatrics* 2004; **114**: 297–316.

Andrew M, Paes B, Johnston M. Development of the hemostatic system in the neonate and young infant. *American Journal of Pediatric Hematology/Oncology* 1990; **12**: 95–104.

Andrew M, Paes B, Milner R, Johnston M, Mitchell L, Tollefsen DM, Castle V, Powers P. Development of the human coagulation system in the healthy premature infant. *Blood* 1988; **72**: 1651–7.

Mou SS, Giroir BP, Molitor-Kirsch EA, et al. Fresh whole blood versus reconstituted blood for pump priming in heart surgery in infants. *New England Journal of Medicine* 2004; **351**: 1635–44.

Northern Neonatal Nursing Initiative (NNNI) Trial Group. A randomized trial comparing the effect of prophylactic intravenous fresh frozen plasma, gelatin or glucose on early mortality and morbidity in preterm babies. *European Journal of Pediatrics* 1996; **155**: 580–8.

Rayment R, Brunskill SJ, Stanworth S, Soothill PW, Roberts DJ, Murphy MF. Antenatal interventions for fetomaternal alloimmune thrombocytopenia. *Cochrane Database of Systematic Reviews* 2005, Issue 1. Art. No. CD004226.

Serious Hazards of Transfusion (SHOT). *Serious Hazards of Transfusion Annual Report 2003*. Manchester, 2004.

CHAPTER 8

Plasma Products and Indications for Their Use

Hannah Cohen and Trevor Baglin

OVERVIEW

- There are few absolute and evidence-based indications for treatment with plasma and plasma products; appropriate use will increase safety.

- Transfusion of cryoprecipitate exposes the patient to multiple donors and therefore fresh frozen plasma (FFP) is recommended for the bleeding associated with the hypofibrinogenaemia of disseminated intravascular coagulation, massive blood transfusion and thrombolytic agents, with cryoprecipitate reserved for instances when fibrinogen levels remain critically low (<1 g/L).

- Viral-inactivated FFP obtained from non-UK areas free of bovine spongiform encephalopathy and variant Creutzfeld–Jakob disease should be used for children under 16 years, patients with thrombotic thrombocytopenic purpura who require repeated infusions of large volumes of FFP, and, when necessary, patients with congenital deficiencies of factor V and XI.

- Recombinant factor VIII and IX concentrates are the products of choice for patients with haemophilia A and B, respectively, and intermediate purity factor VIII for the treatment of moderate to severe von Willebrand's disease. For these disorders and mild factor XI deficiency desmopressin is preferable to plasma-derived products when the effects are equal.

- Recombinant factor VIIa is useful in the management of bleeding in patients with haemophilia who have inhibitory antibodies and it can be used to treat patients with rare congenital platelet disorders.

- Anti-D immunoglobulin prevents primary Rh immunization and haemolytic disease of the newborn.

The concept that the optimal use of plasma is achieved by fractionation is long established and a wide range of products is available for therapeutic use (Figure 8.1). This chapter considers all these products except albumin.

Most therapeutic plasma products are manufactured from pools of plasma derived from many thousands of donations. All donors are individually screened for mandatory microbiological agents (see Chapters 1 and 13) and the plasma products are made by processes that inactivate or remove (or both) any contaminating viruses.

ABC of Transfusion, 4th edition, 2009. Edited by Marcela Contreras. © 2009 Blackwell Publishing, ISBN: 978-1-4051-5646-2.

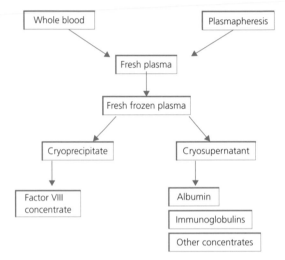

Figure 8.1 Flow diagram of plasma fractionation.

Although the risks of viral transmission are very small, there can never be absolute assurance of freedom from risk. This concern, as well as about that of variant Creutzfeld–Jakob disease (vCJD), has driven the development of recombinant plasma products, and their use has, in some cases, superseded that of plasma-derived products. In the UK, precautions in place to reduce the risk of prion transmission include leucodepletion of all blood components, importation of plasma for fractionation, exclusion of donors who have received a blood transfusion in the UK after 1980, and the use of viral-inactivated fresh frozen plasma (FFP), obtained from non-UK areas free of bovine spongiform encephalopathy (BSE) and vCJD. Such blood products are used for children under 16 years and for patients with thrombotic thrombocytopenic purpura (TTP) who require repeated infusions of large volumes of FFP.

Unpredictable and occasional fatal adverse effects of blood components have been highlighted by the Serious Hazards of Transfusion (SHOT) confidential enquiry (see Chapter 15). Of particular concern are serious allergic reactions and anaphylaxis, and transfusion-related acute lung injury (TRALI): the risk of these acute transfusion reactions is approximately six-fold higher with FFP than with red cell transfusions. Haemolysis from transfused antibodies to blood group antigens, especially A and B, may also occur, usually as a result of 'wrong blood transfusion'. Serious adverse events and reactions related to blood components should be reported to SHOT via the Medicines and Healthcare products Regulatory Agency (MHRA) Serious Adverse Blood Reactions and Events (SABRE) electronic reporting system to meet the requirements of the Blood Safety and Quality Regulations 2005 (see Chapter 20). SHOT also encourages reports on adverse events related to solvent detergent (SD) FFP, although a plasma product, for purposes of comparison with single donor FFP, and on anti-D immunoglobulin. Adverse reactions related to plasma-derived coagulation factors are monitored by the UK Haemophilia Centre Doctors' Organisation (UKHCDO), and those to other plasma fractionated and recombinant products by the MHRA.

It should be appreciated that there are few absolute and evidence-based indications for treatment with plasma and plasma products and that some widely used products are unlicensed and prescribed for a 'named patient' by a 'named doctor'. Especially in acquired disorders, in which sound evidence of efficacy is usually weakest, clinicians should take careful account of the risks of plasma and plasma products before treating patients. Table 8.1 lists the indications for use of different plasma products.

Fresh frozen plasma, cryoprecipitate and cryosupernatant

The indications for the transfusion of FFP, cryoprecipitate and cryosupernatant are very limited. However, although considerable progress has been made in limiting unnecessary transfusion of red cells the use of FFP continues to rise (from 307 804 units in 1999 to 347 882 units in 2005 in the UK). Several audits have shown inappropriate use of FFP, and SHOT data show that acute transfusion reactions have been caused by FFP given inappropriately or for doubtful clinical indications. Current national British Committee for Standards in Haematology (BCSH) guidelines on the appropriate use of FFP, cryoprecipitate and cryosupernatant should be incorporated into local protocols that are readily available in relevant clinical and laboratory areas, included in induction and update training, and subject to clinical audit. Appropriate use of these blood components will increase safety and should be driven in all hospital trusts by the hospital transfusion teams in accordance with the Department of Health circular *Better Blood Transfusion: safe and appropriate use of blood*. The risks of transmitting infection by FFP, cryoprecipitate and cryosupernatant are similar to those of other blood components unless pathogen-reduced plasma is used.

Fresh frozen plasma

The two types of viral-inactivated FFP currently available in the UK are methylene blue and light-treated FFP (MBFFP) and SDFFP (available commercially as Octaplas®) (Figures 8.2–8.4). These products should be used for the treatment of congenital deficiencies of coagulation factors (e.g. factor V) when there is no specific factor concentrate available. Factor XI concentrate administration may be associated with thrombosis and in patients with factor XI deficiency with a history of cardiovascular disease, in whom treatment with desmopressin (see below) is relatively contraindicated, SDFFP should be administered. Used aggressively, with plasma exchange, viral-inactivated FFP which should be viral-inactivated, is essential in the treatment of patients with TTP (see below). BCSH

guidelines on oral anticoagulation recommend prothrombin complex concentrates (two products, Octaplex® and Beriplex® P/N are licensed) rather than FFP for the reversal of the effects of oral anticoagulation associated with serious bleeding.

Despite being widely advocated for patients with multiple coagulation defects, as in disseminated intravascular coagulation (DIC), massive transfusion and liver disease, the effect of FFP is poorly defined. In DIC, FFP is indicated if the patient is bleeding but should not be used if there is no bleeding regardless of the results of laboratory tests. In massive blood transfusion, whilst 'formula replacement' is not recommended, when rapid turnaround of coagulation tests cannot be guaranteed, FFP infusion should be considered after one blood volume is lost. A locally agreed algorithm is essential. What is clear is that, if any benefit is to be obtained, FFP must be given in adequate quantities and rapidly: 12–15 ml/kg (about 1 L for an adult), repeated if necessary, aiming to maintain the PT/APTT (prothrombin time/activated partial thromboplastin time) ratios at <1.5 and fibrinogen at >1.0 g/L. FFP should be used to correct the depletion of coagulation factors in bleeding associated with thrombolysis.

There is no justification for the use of FFP as a volume expander because crystalloids are effective, safer, cheaper and more readily available. Patients likely to receive large or repeated doses of FFP should be offered vaccination against hepatitis A and B and post-transfusion surveillance of hepatitis A, B and C, human immunodeficiency virus (HIV) and parvovirus status.

Cryoprecipitate

Cryoprecipitate is prepared from FFP by slow thawing at $4 \pm 2°C$ (Figure 8.5). The resulting precipitate is then separated from the supernatant and refrozen for storage. Cryoprecipitate contains factor VIII, fibrinogen, von Willebrand factor (vWF), factor XIII and fibronectin in higher concentrations than they are found in plasma, and its preparation is normally the first step in plasma fractionation.

Fibrinogen concentrate (even though it is unlicensed) and factor XIII concentrate (licensed as Fibrogammin®) are preferable to cryoprecipitate in the treatment of congenital hypodys- or hypofibrinogenaemia and factor XIII deficiency, respectively. Transfusion of cryoprecipitate exposes the patient to multiple donors and therefore FFP has been recommended for bleeding associated with the hypofibrinogenaemia of DIC, massive blood transfusion and thrombolytic agents, with cryoprecipitate reserved for instances when fibrinogen levels remain critically low (<1 g/L). One litre of FFP provides on average 2.69 g fibrinogen (range 1.54–5.00), while an adult therapeutic dose (two pools) of cryoprecipitate provides, on average, 4 g fibrinogen (range 0.54–3.79), in a volume of 320–340 ml (R. Cardigan, personal communication). As a result, a rise in fibrinogen can be achieved more rapidly with cryoprecipitate than with FFP infusion; therefore – particularly in massive obstetric haemorrhage where profound hypofibrinogenaemia may occur – cryoprecipitate should be given 'sooner rather than later'.

Cryosupernatant

This is the supernatant plasma removed during the preparation of cryoprecipitate (see below).

Table 8.1 Plasma product concentrates: indications for use.

Plasma product/recombinant concentrate	Indications for use
Recombinant factor VIII	Congenital deficiency (haemophilia A)
Recombinant factor IX	Congenital deficiency (haemophilia B)
Recombinant factor VIIa	Inhibitors in patients with haemophilia A and B Congenital deficiency of factor VII Congenital platelet disorders ?Uncontrolled bleeding states (trauma or surgery)
Prothrombin complex concentrates (PCC)	Congenital deficiencies of factor II and X Reversal of oral anticoagulation Inhibitors, especially to factor VIII ?Severe liver disease
Activated prothrombin complex concentrates (PCC)	Inhibitors, especially to factor VIII
Porcine factor VIII (recombinant product undergoing clinical trials)	Factor VIII inhibitors
Intermediate purity factor VIII concentrate	Congenital deficiency (moderate/severe von Willebrand's disease)
8Y (intermediate purity factor VIII concentrate)	Congenital deficiency (ADAMTS 13 in thrombotic thrombocytopenic purpura)
Factor VII	Congenital deficiency Reversal of oral anticoagulation associated with severe bleeding (NB Octaplex® and Beriplex® P/N (licensed PCCs) contains factor VII) ?Severe liver disease
Factor XI	Congenital deficiency (desmopressin is an alternative but viral-inactivated FFP is preferable in patients with a history of cardiovascular disease)
Fibrinogen	Congenital hypo- and dysfibrinogenaemia
Factor XIII	Congenital deficiency
Fibrin sealant/glue	Congenital and acquired haemostatic disorders to promote local haemostasis
Antithrombin (a recombinant product, ATryn®, is licensed (pan-European) for prophylaxis of venous thromboembolism in patients with congenital antithrombin deficiency undergoing surgery)	Congenital deficiency ?Disseminated intravascular coagulation ?Liver transplantation ?Other acquired deficiency states
Protein C	Congenital deficiency ?Meningococcal purpura fulminans
Recombinant activated protein C	Severe sepsis
Alpha-1 antitrypsin	Hereditary deficiency (emphysema, cirrhosis)
CI esterase inhibitor	Hereditary angioedema
Fibronectin	?Acquired deficiency states
Intravenous immunoglobulin (IVIg)	Congenital ahypo- and hypogammaglobulinaemia Chronic lymphocytic leukaemia Immune thrombocytopenic purpura ?Other acquired immune disorders
Anti-D (usually intramuscular)	Prevention of primary RhD immunization and haemolytic disease of the newborn
Anti-D (intravenous)	Refractory idiopathic thrombocytopenic purpura

Plasma exchange

To date, the only condition where FFP is recommended as replacement fluid for PEX is acute TTP, where intensive PEX remains the mainstay of therapy, reducing mortality rates from >90% to 10–20%. Patients with TTP have deficiency or inhibition of ADAMTS 13 (vWF-cleaving protease), a metalloprotease that normally cleaves ultralarge vWF multimers released from the vascular endothelium. The resultant accumulation of ultralarge vWF multimers in TTP (Figure 8.6) leads to platelet activation and aggregation, which in turn leads to microvascular occlusion by

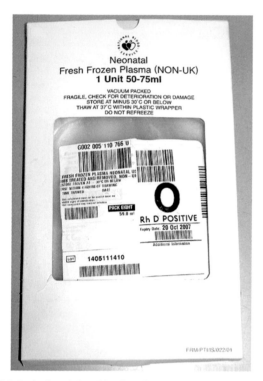

Figure 8.2 Pack of methylene blue fresh frozen plasma for neonates.

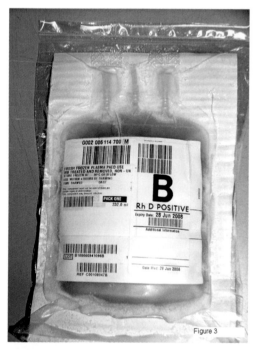

Figure 8.3 Pack of methylene blue fresh frozen plasma for paediatric use.

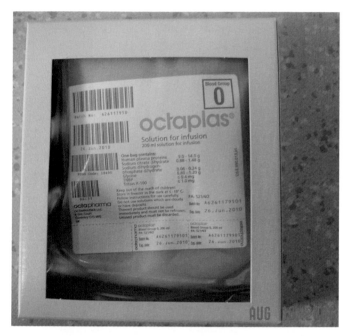

Figure 8.4 Pack of solvent detergent fresh frozen plasma (Octaplas®).

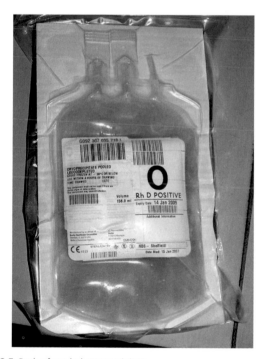

Figure 8.5 Pack of pooled cryoprecipitate.

platelet-rich thrombi and ischaemic organ damage. Despite the documented low incidence of TTP in the UK these patients use 20–25% of national plasma stocks. The Department of Health has recommended that replacement in PEX for TTP should be with SDFFP in adults and with MBFFP in children under 16 years. Preliminary studies suggest that SDFFP, which, unlike standard FFP, lacks high molecular weight vWF multimers, may be more effective than standard FFP or MBFFP in TTP. The use of cryosupernatant has now been superseded as it does not appear to be more effective than standard FFP. Of note, SDFFP has been associated with venous thromboembolism, possibly due to acquired protein S deficiency, when used as replacement for PEX in TTP. Low molecular weight heparin thromboprophylaxis should therefore be instituted when the platelet count rises to $>50 \times 10^9$/L. In addition, patients should be fitted with graduated elastic compression stockings and care should be taken with indwelling lines, particularly to avoid

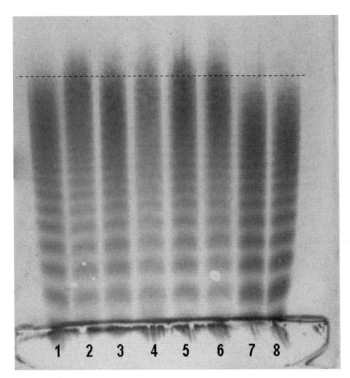

Figure 8.6 Ultralarge von Willebrand factor (vWF) multimers in patients with thrombotic thrombocytopenic purpura can be seen on sodium dodecyl sulfate polyacrylamide gel electrophoresis (SDS-PAGE) in lanes 2–6 above the dotted line (with normal vWF multimers in lanes 1, 7 and 8).

Table 8.2 Half-lives of infused coagulation factors contained in fresh frozen plasma.

Factor		Half life of infused factor (hours)*
I	(fibrinogen)	72–120
II	(prothrombin)	72
V	(proaccelerin)	12
VII	(proconvertin)	2–5
VIII	(antihaemophiliac factor)	8–12
IX	(Christmas factor)	12–18
X	(Stuart–Prower factor)	24–40
XI	(plasma thromboplastin antecedent)	60–80
XII	(Hageman's factor)	40–50
XIII	(fibrin stabilizing factor)	216–240
Antithrombin		24–60
Protein C		6–8
Protein S		12–60
Fibronectin		24–72

*Half-lives of coagulation factors may be shortened when there is increased consumption, for example in disseminated intravascular coagulation, after surgery or during thrombotic episodes.

infection. Concerns have been raised about the efficacy of MBFFP as replacement in PEX for TTP as more PEX procedures may be required. Currently, methylene blue cryosupernatant is unavailable in the UK.

The optimal regimen for PEX is undefined, but the current recommendation is for at least 1.0 plasma volume exchange daily until at least 2 days after remission is achieved (defined as normal neurology, platelets $>150 \times 10^9$/L, normal lactate dehydrogenase levels, and rising haemoglobin concentration). More intensive PEX (twice daily or daily 1.5 volume exchanges) may be useful in patients with severe acute neurological or cardiological manifestations.

Recently, the monoclonal CD20 antibody rituximab, used initially as second line therapy in patients with refractory TTP, has been associated with prompt remission and a reduction in the number of PEX required.

Factor VIII and IX concentrates

Factor VIII and IX concentrates are the products of choice for patients with haemophilia A (factor VIII deficiency) who do not respond adequately to desmopressin (1-deamino-8-D-arginine vasopressin, DDAVP, see below) and for patients with haemophilia B (factor IX deficiency). Patients with factor VIII levels of less than 0.10 IU/ml are unlikely to respond adequately to DDAVP and require factor replacement. Patients with factor IX deficiency

do not respond to DDAVP therapy. In the UK recombinant factors VIII and IX are now recommended, as there is no associated risk of transmission of human-borne infectious disease. Factor concentrates are supplied as freeze-dried powders that are reconstituted with a small volume of sterile water before intravenous injection.

Factor VIII has a short half-life (about 8–12 hours *in vivo*) (Table 8.2), so twice-daily repeated injections are necessary for a sustained effect. Injection of 1 IU/kg of factor VIII concentrate will raise the plasma factor VIII level by approximately 0.02 IU/ml. Factor IX has a longer half-life (about 12–18 hours) and once-daily injections may be adequate for a sustained effect. Injection of 1 IU/kg of factor IX concentrate will raise the plasma factor IX level by approximately 0.01 IU/ml. For example, to raise the factor level by 0.30 IU/ml (a normal level is >0.50 IU/ml) in a 50 kg male would require 750 units of factor VIII or 1500 units of factor IX concentrate.

The minimum level of factor VIII required for treatment of bleeding has not been determined from randomized clinical trials. Early mild haemarthrosis is often treated with a single infusion of factor concentrate to raise the plasma level to 0.15–0.20 IU/ml. More severe haemarthrosis requires repeated infusions and higher plasma levels (0.30–0.50 IU/ml). Intracranial bleeding requires normalization of factor levels with treatment for at least 2–4 weeks to achieve peak plasma levels of 1.0–1.50 IU/ml and troughs not less than 0.50 IU/ml. Treatment to cover surgery requires normalization of factor levels for 7–14 days depending on the type of surgery. Primary prophylaxis with factor concentrate two or three times weekly at doses to keep the trough factor level above 0.01 IU/ml reduces bleeding and hence chronic haemophilic arthropathy. Pharmacokinetic studies are used to optimize dosing schedules for individual patients. With the increased safety of coagulation factor replacement products, prophylaxis has become the preferred treatment option in the UK for males with severe haemophilia. Programmes are typically initiated in the second or third year of life, so an indwelling venous access device (portacath) is often necessary.

Recombinant factor VIII preparations do not contain vWF and are not effective for the treatment of moderate to severe von Willebrand's disease. Intermediate purity products are used to treat moderate to severe von Willebrand's disease. Both high and intermediate purity plasma-derived factor VIII concentrates are available but are no longer used in the UK for treatment of haemophilia A. However, many patients with haemophilia were treated with these products before the availability of recombinant products. Despite the excellent safety record of virally inactivated plasma-derived concentrates it is acknowledged that current viral-inactivation techniques may fail to eliminate all virus transmission by non-lipid-enveloped viruses such as parvovirus. There is no evidence that vCJD can be transmitted by non-cellular blood products but there has been recent anxiety about the theoretical possibility that plasma-derived products could have been contaminated. So far, there have been no documented cases of transmission of vCJD by plasma-derived factor concentrates.

Recombinant factor VIIa

Approximately one-quarter of patients with severe haemophilia A develop an inhibitory immunoglobulin G (IgG) antibody to factor VIII. On average this is detectable after about 10 treatment exposures, and while the antibody is transitory in 50% of patients in the remainder it is permanent unless eradicated by immune-tolerance therapy employing daily high dose factor VIII until the antibody is eliminated. While the antibody is present infused factor VIII is immediately neutralized, and this therapy is ineffective. For such patients, treatment with a 'bypassing agent' is required. High dose recombinant factor VIIa (90 µg/kg/dose) generates thrombin in the absence of either factor VIII or IX and is used to treat bleeding in patients with inhibitors. Typically, up to three treatments at 2-hourly intervals are used. Recombinant factor VIIa can also be used to treat bleeding in patients with haemophilia B with inhibitor antibodies to factor IX, but these occur in less than 1% of such patients. Recombinant factor VIIa can also be used to treat patients with factor VII deficiency and the rare congenital platelet disorders Glanzmann's thrombasthenia and Bernard Soulier syndrome. Recombinant VIIa is not licensed for the treatment of uncontrollable bleeding states following trauma or during major surgery.

Prothrombin complex concentrates

Prothrombin complex concentrates (PCCs) are plasma-derived intermediate purity products containing coagulation factors IX, X and II, and sometimes factor VII. They are used for the reversal of severe overanticoagulation and/or bleeding due to treatment with vitamin K antagonists (mainly warfarin in the UK). They are also used for the treatment of the severe rare bleeding disorders of factor X and factor II deficiency.

Prothrombin complex concentrates are now being used in patients with liver failure although this was previously considered a contraindication to their use. In liver disease PCCs can correct only part of the overall haemostatic abnormality, and carry a risk of provoking DIC. DIC can also occur in patients without liver disease who are treated with repeated doses of PCCs.

Activated PCCs are used as 'bypassing agents', as an alternative to recombinant factor VIIa, for the treatment of patients with severe haemophilia with an inhibitor.

Other coagulation factor concentrates

Other coagulation factor concentrates (factor XIII, fibrinogen, factor XI) have been produced by fractionation but are not always available. Currently a factor XIII concentrate (Fibrogammin®) is available in the UK for the treatment of patients with severe factor XIII deficiency. Some concentrates of fibrinogen or factor XI that were previously available were associated with a significant risk of thrombosis. At present viral-inactivated FFP is typically used for the treatment of patients with factor XI deficiency. Concentrates of natural anticoagulants, antithrombin and protein C are occasionally used in patients with congenital, and sometimes acquired, deficiencies of specific anticoagulants, for example protein C concentrate for purpura fulminans. A recombinant activated protein C concentrate is licensed for the treatment of severe sepsis. A recombinant antithrombin product (ATryn®) is licensed (pan-European) for prophylaxis of venous thromboembolism in patients with congenital antithrombin deficiency undergoing surgery.

Desmopressin (DDAVP), a synthetic analogue of the non-apeptide arginine vasopressin, can lead to a marked increase in blood levels of factor VIII and vWF. In patients with mild haemophilia A and von Willebrand's disease DDAVP is effective in the treatment of bleeding episodes and to cover surgery. DDAVP may also be useful in patients with mild factor XI deficiency. DDAVP has a similar effect to cryoprecipitate in the treatment of the bleeding tendency in chronic renal failure, where a functional defect in vWF–platelet interaction appears to play a role in the abnormal haemostasis observed.

For all indications DDAVP is clearly preferable to plasma-derived products for reasons of both cost and safety when the effect is equal. DDAVP should be used with caution in elderly individuals and pregnant women, and avoided in those with evidence of arterio-vascular disease. In young children, precautions should be taken to prevent fluid overloading and hyponatraemia, and DDAVP should probably be avoided in children under 2 years old.

Immunoglobulins

Specific immunoglobulins

Specific immunoglobulins are obtained from donors whose plasma contains selected high titre IgG antibodies, as a result either of previous infection or of active immunization. Usually given by intramuscular injection, preparations are available for use in the

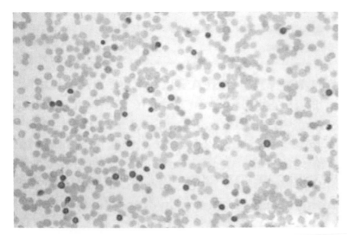

Figure 8.7 Fetal cells (darkly stained) in the maternal circulation of a RhD-negative woman as shown by the Kleihauer (acid elution) technique. A 500 IU intramuscular dose of anti-D immunoglobulin is sufficient for 4 ml of red cells. If a fetomaternal haemorrhage of >4 ml is indicated by the Kleihauer test, the volume of fetomaternal haemorrhage must be confirmed by flow cytometry and an adequate dose of anti-D administered (larger doses may be given intravenously) to prevent primary Rh immunization and haemolytic disease of the newborn.

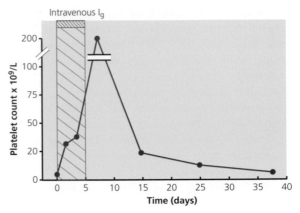

Figure 8.8 Time course of a typical response of platelets to high doses of intravenous immunoglobulin (Ig) in adult (chronic) idiopathic thrombocytopenic purpura.

passive prophylaxis of varicella-zoster, tetanus, hepatitis B and other infections. Immunity lasts a few weeks. Anti-D immunoglobulin, usually given intramuscularly, is used in the prevention of primary Rh immunization and haemolytic disease of the newborn (see Chapter 6) (Figure 8.7), and intravenous anti-D in refractory idiopathic thrombocytopenic purpura (ITP).

Intravenous anti-D in ITP is suitable as second line therapy for RhD-positive patients who are not splenectomized (it is rarely effective in splenectomized patients and therefore not recommended). The mechanism of action is believed to be mediated through the destruction of RhD-positive red cells, which are preferentially removed by the reticuloendothelial system, particularly the spleen, thus sparing autoantibody-coated platelets through Fcγ receptor blockade. The effect on the platelet count tends to last for only a few weeks. Common toxicities of anti-D include fever/chill reactions, which can be ameliorated by pretreatment with corticosteroids, and extravascular haemolysis; the risk of this is lessened by avoiding treatment in those with a positive direct antiglobulin test unless attributable to prior intravenous Ig or anti-D Ig therapy.

Non-specific immunoglobulin

Non-specific ('normal') immunoglobulin is derived from the pooled plasma of non-selected donors and contains antibodies to all the viruses prevalent in the donor population. One of the main indications for its intramuscular use is in the passive prophylaxis of hepatitis A. Preparations made for intravenous use have the advantage that much larger doses may be given with minimal discomfort to the patient.

Intravenous Ig was introduced primarily for replacement therapy in patients with congenital hypogammaglobulinaemia, but its range of application has now broadened considerably to include replacement in acquired hypogammaglobulinaemia as seen in chronic lymphocytic leukaemia, and in immunomodulation, especially in some autoimmune disorders. Intravenous Ig is useful in patients with ITP when the platelet count has to be raised rapidly because of bleeding, or prior to intervention likely to induce bleeding. The usual dosage, a total of 2 g/kg over 2–5 days, elevates the platelet count in 75% of patients with ITP, 50% of whom achieve normal counts, but the responses are transient, lasting up to 3–4 weeks (Figure 8.8). Its mode of action is not certain but probably includes blockade of Fc receptors on macrophages or other effectors of antibody-dependent cytotoxicity. Intravenous Ig has an excellent safety record although renal impairment or failure have been reported. These products are often used for unlicensed indications, including a variety of autoimmune neurological conditions, in the absence of any prospective, evidence-based clinical trial data.

Other plasma products

Several other plasma products are available, and there is little doubt that these concentrates can be effective in raising subnormal concentrations of circulating plasma factors. Except in rare congenital deficiency states, however, convincing evidence of clinical benefit is generally weak and indications remain ill defined.

Acknowledgments

The authors are grateful to Professor Sam J. Machin for critical review of this chapter.

Further reading

Allford SL, Hunt BJ, Rose P, Machin SJ. Guidelines on the diagnosis and management of the thrombotic microangiopathic haemolytic anaemias. *British Journal of Haematology* 2003; **120**: 556–73.

Baglin TP, Keeling DM, Watson HG. Guidelines on oral anticoagulation (warfarin): third edition – 2005 update. *British Journal of Haematology* 2006; **132**: 277–85.

British Committee for Standards in Haematology (BCSH) Blood Transfusion Task Force. Guidelines for the use of fresh frozen plasma, cryoprecipitate and cryosupernatant. *British Journal of Haematology* 2004; **126**: 11–28.

Health Service circular. *Better Blood Transfusion: safe and appropriate use of blood.* Series No. 2007/001, Gateway reference 9058. Department of Health, London, 2007.

Stainsby D, MacLennan S, Thomas D, Isaac J, Hamilton PJ. Guidelines on the management of massive blood loss. *British Journal of Haematology* 2006; 135; 635–41.

UK Haemophilia Centre Doctors' Organisation (UKHCDO). UKHCDO guidelines on the selection and use of therapeutic products to treat haemophilia and other hereditary bleeding disorders. *Haemophilia* 2003; **9**: 1–23.

CHAPTER 9

Human Albumin Solutions and the Controversy of Crystalloids Versus Colloids

Neil Soni

OVERVIEW

- Albumin is available as 4.5% isotonic and 20% hypertonic solutions.
- Serum albumin falls rapidly in many disease states. In acute states the rapid fall is often due to redistribution.
- Low serum albumin is a prognostic indicator in many chronic disease states.
- There are many indications, although few have an adequate evidence base.
- Suggestions that albumin is unsafe were clearly refuted in a large clinical trial, SAFE, but specific areas where albumin may be of particular benefit or be detrimental have not yet been delineated.

Table 9.1 Composition of albumin solutions.

	4.5% albumin (500 ml bottle)	20% albumin (100 ml bottle)
Albumin (human), approx.	45 g/L (22.5 g)	200 g/L (20 g)
Colloid oncotic pressure	26–30 mmHg	100–120 mmHg
Sodium	120–160 mmol/L	70–160 mmol/L
Potassium	<2 mmol/L	<10 mmol/L
Stabilizers vary Sodium-*n*-octanote, mmol/L Sodium acetyl tryptanoate		
Bottle size	250 or 500ml	50 or 100 ml

Albumin as a solution is available in two basic formats. The first is 4.5% albumin solution, which is essentially isotonic with an ion distribution not dissimilar to plasma, and the second is 20% albumin, which is a hypertonic solution. It is often described as 'salt-poor albumin' as the ratio of sodium to albumin is approximately 25% of that in the 4.5% solution (Table 9.1).

The preparation of human albumin is by two pasteurization processes, effective against enveloped viruses such as human immunodeficiency virus (HIV), hepatitis B virus (HBV), hepatitis C virus (HCV) and non-enveloped viruses such as hepatitis A. Both the ethanol fractionation and heat treatment processes may have effects on the molecular structure, in particular the charge, which may then influence properties such as binding. At present UK supplies are derived from US plasma because of anxiety about prions (variant Creutzfeldt–Jakob disease or vCJD).

Physiology of albumin

Human albumin is a polypeptide with a molecular weight of 66 248. It is a small molecule (compared with fibrinogen, with a molecular weight of 340 000, or immunoglobulin G, with a molecular weight of 150 000) and is synthesized in hepatocytes at a rate of 9–12 g

per day in an adult. It is highly soluble and has a strong net negative charge. There are many variants of albumin. It is predominantly an extravascular protein with more albumin in the interstitium than intravascularly, although at a lower concentration.

There is a normal circulation of albumin from the intravascular to interstitial spaces, with return via the lymphatic vessels.

Clinical properties of albumin

Albumin is strongly charged and has at least four discrete binding sites, which can bind reversibly to cations and anions and a wide range of other molecules including drugs (Table 9.2). Alterations in the quantity or structure of albumin will affect competitive binding and hence drug levels.

Albumin represents 75–80% of the plasma colloid osmotic pressure (COP). It is thus the major determinant of the plasma and interstitial COP component in Starling's equation for fluid flux across the capillary wall. The relative role of albumin alters in severe illness as the profile of plasma proteins changes. Acid–base balance is influenced by the concentration of albumin. Free radical scavenging is possible because of its thiol groups. Administered albumin will act as a 'donor' of thiol groups, and rejuvenate other intravascular proteins by donating electrons. It also has an anticoagulant and antithrombotic function. Albumin reputedly has a protective effect on membrane permeability but this is controversial.

ABC of Transfusion, 4th edition, 2009. Edited by Marcela Contreras. © 2009 Blackwell Publishing, ISBN: 978-1-4051-5646-2.

Table 9.2 Some ions, cations and molecules that bind to albumin.

Calcium, copper, silver, mercury

Amino acids

Fatty acids

Thyroxine

Glucose, galactose

Warfarin, phenytoin, diazepam, non-steroidal anti-inflammatories, digoxin and many others

Table 9.3 Illness and low serum albumin.

Cause of low albumin	Mechanisms/implications
Analbuminaemia	No synthesis. No major clinical effects
Starvation	Rapid reduction in albumin synthesis. Poor specific marker of nutrition, but rapid turnover proteins such as prealbumin are better nutritional markers. Associated with poor outcome
Liver disease	Largely caused by redistribution but also catabolism and synthesis. It is not a strong specific synthesis marker
Renal disease	Leakage in albuminuria and nephrosis. Also falls with dialysis
Pre-eclampsia	Due to redistribution, not synthesis
Malignancy	Reduced synthesis, and increased catabolism and redistribution. Cytokine activity also implicated (commonly tumour necrosis factor). Associated with poor prognosis
Stress response	Synthesis of acute phase proteins increases. Albumin may decrease (not confirmed)
Burns	Catabolism, massive leak from site and redistribution. Reduction in synthesis
Trauma	Stress response. Redistribution and catabolism
Surgery	Stress response. Redistribution
Sepsis	Redistribution, with later catabolism and reduced synthesis

Clinical associations of serum albumin

The serum albumin concentration often falls in disease states and it is important to differentiate the meaning of the serum albumin value in relatively stable, albeit chronic, states and the rapidly changing values found in acute severe illness. In chronic states, serum concentration reflects the balance of synthesis and catabolism; in acute states, concentration may be significantly influenced by both these. The predominant cause of the concentration change is redistribution. Low serum albumin is seen in many disease states (Table 9.3; Figures 9.1 and 9.2).

Preoperative hypoalbuminaemia may be a marker of malnutrition and is a predictor of poor outcome.

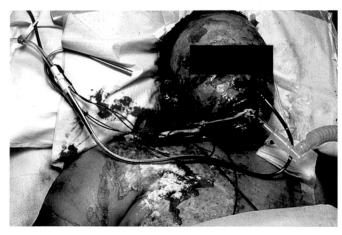

Figure 9.1 This patient sustained severe burns to the head and neck, back, arms, chest and abdomen in a road traffic accident. With an excess of 70% burns, he had a massive fluid requirement on admission, but also recurrent requirements during debridement and grafting. Although he demonstrated hypoalbuminaemia as a consequence of both albumin loss and distribution, many units do not electively replace albumin but rather use nutritional support.

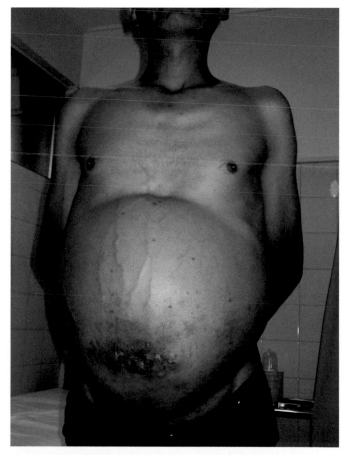

Figure 9.2 This patient shows several of the clinical features of cirrhotic liver failure with portal hypertension. He has obvious ascites, collateral veins in the abdominal wall, and possibly some muscle wasting. With this degree of liver failure it is likely that he is hypoalbuminaemic, but he is clearly active and mobile so albumin replacement is not indicated.

Prognostic value of serum albumin

In the relatively 'steady state' of severe chronic illness (i.e. not acute and fulminant), a reduced serum albumin is a relatively reliable marker of the severity of illness and is associated with a poor outcome in many disease states (Table 9.4).

Table 9.4 Low serum albumin has been shown to be associated with poor outcome in the following specific diseases and conditions.

AIDS (acquired immune deficiency syndrome)/*Pneumocystis carinii* pneumonia	Lung cancer
	Lymphoma
	Malignant melanoma
Bone marrow transplant	Myeloma
Breast cancer	Ovarian cancer
Burns	Pancreatic cancer
Clostridium difficile colitis	Pancreatitis
Colorectal cancer	Pneumonia
Gastric cancer	Pre-eclampsia
Juvenile rheumatoid arthritis	Renal conditions:
Leukaemia	continuous ambulatory
Liver conditions:	glomerulonephritis
alcoholic cirrhosis	peritoneal dialysis
cholangiocarcinoma	renal failure
hepatitis B cirrhosis	Ulcerative colitis
hepatocellular cancer	
post shunt	
primary biliary cirrhosis	
pyogenic abscess	

Indications

There are many indications for the use of albumin, including hypovolaemia and hypoalbuminaemia (see Table 9.5 for the more common indications). The former needs no explanation, but the latter is a consequence of being able to measure the serum concentration and to have the material available with which to correct the value.

As an unfortunate consequence of the association between albumin value and disease outcome it has been impossible to separate the indications for albumin from the influence of those associations. A low serum albumin, which may be a marker of illness, nutritional state or of redistribution, has often been treated with albumin infusions to attempt to change the measured value in the hope that a corrected value would influence the disease state underlying it. This is reflected in its usage and in its variable efficacy. In Table 9.5 there is a column called efficacy that indicates if the specific indication is considered effective or not. In many of the indications there is widespread use but little evidence for specific efficacy (Aboulghar et al. 2002; Barron et al. 2004; Maitland et al. 2005).

It is quite clear from Table 9.5 that there are a large number of indications where there is a lack of evidence of benefit from the treatment. These need exploration, as do those with some evidence of benefit. The use of albumin in primary peritonitis and in children with falciparum malaria are both indications with at least one study conferring benefit, but in both this needs confirmation. The Saline versus Albumin Fluid Evaluation (SAFE) study (see below),

Table 9.5 Indications for albumin use.

Solution	General indication	Specific indication	Efficacy
Colloid 4.5%	Intravascular volume replacement	Hypovolaemia	Yes
		Paracentesis in liver failure	Probable
		Primary peritonitis in liver failure	Probable
	Support colloid oncotic pressure		No
	Support serum albumin	Non-specific: transport membrane integrity, coagulation, to prevent ileus	?
		Protein-losing entero/nephropathy	? Some advocates
		Nutrition	No
	Therapeutic plasma exchange		It is used
	Ovarian hyperstimulation syndrome	At time of oocyte collection Mechanism unknown	Yes/maybe
	To treat metabolic acidosis	Use as a buffer	? Used in neonates
	To treat falciparum malaria with acidosis in children	Used as volume replacement	Yes, reduced mortality
Hypertonic solution/ colloid 20%	Intravascular volume replacement		Yes
	Fluid redistribution	Renal dialysis and to initiate diuresis	Some advocates
		Acute lung injury: fluid redistribution, to initiate diuresis	Some advocates.
	Ovarian hyperstimulation syndrome	Intravascular volume	Yes/maybe

Table 9.6 SAFE subgroup analyses: area of focus and relative risk (RR) of mortality and confidence intervals (CI) when using albumin versus saline as fluid resuscitation therapy.

Focus area	RR and CI of using albumin versus saline	Benefit/disadvantage
Trauma with head injury	RR: 1.62 95% CI: 1.12–2.34 $P = 0.009$	Possible detriment from albumin
Trauma without head injury	RR: 1.00 95% CI: 0.56–1.79 $P = 1.00$	No difference
Severe sepsis	RR: 0.87 95% CI: 0.74–1.02 $P = 0.09$	Possible advantage to albumin

Table 9.7 Considerations when using colloids.

- Colloids may require less total volume to have the same volume expansion effect. Benefit?
- Crystalloids are cheap
- Coagulation: colloids may affect coagulation. Antithrombotic effects of dextran and hydroxyethyl starch
- Clearance: starch may stay in the reticuloendothelial system
- Renal failure: hydroxyethyl starch and albumin may increase the risk of acute renal failure. There is evidence this may be a problem with higher molecular weight starch
- Head injury: colloids, specifically albumin, may have adverse effects (not confirmed)
- Disease states where albumin may be of benefit: paediatric falciparum malaria, primary peritonitis and severe sepsis

which was designed to evaluate any mortality outcome difference between albumin and saline when used for fluid resuscitation in the critically ill, showed no difference in overall mortality although there were some interesting trends in the subgroup analysis (Finfer et al. 2004). These pose some new questions about potential indications and contraindications (Table 9.6). These all need further targeted study and cannot at present be seen as either indications or contraindications.

The crystalloid/colloid controversy and the suggestion that the use of albumin is associated with a higher mortality

The use of intravenous fluids to support the intravascular compartment in the management of hypovolaemia is well established. The two main classes of fluids are crystalloids and colloids. The principal difference is that the latter contain larger molecules and are therefore expected to stay in the intravascular compartment longer. Crystalloids are relatively free to move between compartments and will leave the intravascular space and distribute into the interstitium. Therefore it seems likely that colloid is more efficient than crystalloid, requiring a smaller volume to achieve a sustained effect, and in normal physiological circumstances this is true. In clinical circumstances normal physiology becomes pathophysiology and the situation changes. Fluid tends to redistribute far more readily and so do some larger molecules. Colloid efficacy is reduced, but for volume expansion it is still more efficient than crystalloid and it is this concept that underpins the argument about which is better.

Crystalloids are cheap, easy to use and effective. Even though large volumes may be required, the fluid will come back out as easily as it went in. Apart from fluid overload, which applies equally to colloids, specific complications are few. Excess saline can cause acidosis.

Colloids are more expensive and more effective, and smaller volumes are required to achieve the same effect, although once the larger molecules move into the interstitium there are those that worry about how they get back out later. Specific complications include a low incidence of anaphylactoid and anaphylactic reactions, potential alterations in coagulation, and the potential, although minor, risk of transmission of infectious agents in the human-derived products. There also appears to be a difference in propensity to acute renal failure in severe sepsis between the colloids: the gelatins have a possible benefit over starches or albumin (Schortgen et al. 2001). There are some general points to consider when deciding on colloid use (Table 9.7).

Both crystalloids and colloids have proponents, and the longevity of the debate is a clear indication of the lack of hard evidence that either is advantageous.

Albumin is a colloid and was considered the gold standard. It is present in plasma and has multiple physiological functions; it can be measured and in illness is almost always at a lower level than normal, implying a deficit. There is a well known association between low serum albumin values and outcome, so the scene is set for this colloid not only to be effective as a volume expanding agent but to have a myriad of other benefits.

The controversy has been on two fronts. The first was whether colloids are better than crystalloids, and the second was which colloid is best, given that the alternative colloids to albumin are all synthetic and devoid of potential physiological benefits beyond plasma expansion. The information currently available refers to those colloid solutions that are readily available and have been tested (Table 9.8). Balanced salt solutions, as carriers for colloids, are now available and it has been suggested that they may be beneficial, adding a new dimension to the debate. It seems logical to put colloid into a more balanced solution and, although there is some evidence to support this idea, more information is needed (Vercueil et al. 2005).

In summary there is a large amount of opinion but no hard evidence that there is a real difference in outcome either between crystalloids and colloids or between crystalloids and albumin. A new study or studies that could clearly show a difference was needed and it was into this scenario that two systematic reviews from the Cochrane Collaboration appeared, both in the *British Medical Journal*, within a relatively short time period (Cochrane Injuries Group Albumin Reviewers 1998; Schierhout & Roberts

Table 9.8 Available colloids.

Colloid	Characteristics	Problems
Albumin 4.5%	Isotonic	Cost Hypotension: rare
Albumin 20%	Hyperoncotic Relatively salt poor	Expensive
Gelatins	MW 30 000 to 5000 Shorter intravascular effect Excreted through kidney	Allergy: rare
Dextrans (complex polysaccharide)	Has anticoagulant effect MW ranges from 30 000 to 150 000 Complex polysaccharides	Allergy: rare Anticoagulant effect Nephrotoxicity rare Mechanism unknown
Starches	Wide range of characteristics MW 200 000 to 450 000 Long half-life in plasma	Larger MW starches affect coagulation Remains in reticuloendothelial system Itching
Balanced colloid	Starch in a more physiological electrolyte solution Potentially better in terms of less acidosis	

MW, molecular weight.

1998). In essence, they showed that both colloids and albumin were associated with a higher mortality than crystalloids. In the new era of evidence-based medicine – with systematic reviews becoming a gold standard akin to a randomized controlled trial – these studies had a profound effect in terms of evidence credibility. They were not the first meta-analyses, but a previous analysis by Velanovich (1989), showing an advantage in the use of colloids in trauma, had not been generally noticed. There was a call to review practice and the net effect was a significant deepening of the entire controversy.

Subsequent meta-analyses have failed to find the same outcome. One analysis pointed out that a randomized controlled trial almost three times the size of the meta-analysis would be needed to produce adequate power for a conclusion. There was widespread criticism of the studies. These criticisms were based on the numbers, population heterogeneity, treatment heterogeneity, and the time period studied during which fluid management had altered considerably, as well as other aspects of these reviews. The real benefit from these publications was that they triggered a massive randomized controlled trial involving 6997 patients in Australia and New Zealand. This was the SAFE study mentioned above. It tested the use of saline against albumin for fluid resuscitation in the critically ill (Finfer et al. 2004); there was no difference in outcome. The lack of concordance between this well executed trial and the earlier meta-analyses casts further doubt on the validity of the latter. Since the initial report subgroup analysis has become available (see Table 9.6), and this has highlighted questions about specific clinical areas of use.

More recent Cochrane Collaboration updates have stated that 'there is no evidence that albumin reduces mortality in critically ill patients with burns and hypoalbuminaemia'. Interestingly, the areas not yet tested by large trials and therefore dependent on meta-analysis, such as burns and hypoalbuminaemia, are still reported as indicating an increased risk, based on the meta-analysis of a few small trials; however, there is no comment on the validity of the statement (Alderson et al. 2004). Paradoxically, the use of albumin fell during this time period as obvious benefits over other colloids were hard to find, while the cost issues in most countries mitigated in favour of synthetic colloids.

The current position is therefore that the colloid/crystalloid debate will continue. The only irrefutable fact is that crystalloids are cheaper, and while there is no clear advantage in the use of albumin over other colloids the obvious disadvantage of albumin is cost.

The controversy has been beneficial as it has established that there is limited information about an 'everyday' management issue. Further work is needed to identify real benefits or real problems, if they exist, from the use of colloids rather than crystalloids. Albumin has never been tested adequately in specific disease states to ascertain if the potential physiological benefits can be realized. In some disease states such as paediatric falciparum malaria there is significant evidence to suggest possible benefit. In others, such as primary peritonitis, the trial that demonstrated benefit from albumin compared albumin with nothing. This trial needs to be repeated to determine if the effect was from albumin or from volume replacement. Likewise, in areas such as head injury the possibility of detriment needs to be clarified.

There is a dearth of information in hypoalbuminaemia about the effects of reduced binding capability, the reduction in thiol groups for scavenging, or even the role in acid–base balance. The gross heterogeneity of the critically ill as a population makes this group a difficult one to study. Investigation should target specific areas of use if benefits are to be identified. The information available hints that benefit may be found in disease states where the serum albumin is low from depletion as well as distribution. This needs to be explored. In other situations, such as head injury, there is a suggestion that albumin, and therefore by default other members of the colloid group, might have detrimental effects. This information desperately needs clarifying.

Conclusion

There are no overwhelming benefits from any one volume expander. Serum albumin is a non-specific marker of disease associated with poor outcome. It is a simple matter of cause and effect. Low albumin is the effect and treating it does not reverse the cause. Research into any specific benefits of crystalloids and each type of colloid is long overdue.

Acknowledgments

The author would like to thank Simon Finfer for his advice and help in preparing this chapter. Dr Cristina Martinez is thanked for providing figure 9.2.

Further reading

Aboulghar M, Evers JH, Al-Inany H. Intravenous albumin for preventing severe ovarian hyperstimulation syndrome: a Cochrane review. *Human Reproduction* 2002; **17**(12): 3027–32.

Alderson P, Bunn F, Lefebvre C, Li WP, Li L, Roberts I, Schierhout G. Human albumin solution for resuscitation and volume expansion in critically ill patients. *Cochrane Database of Systematic Reviews* 2004; **4**: CD001208.

Barron ME, Wilkes MM, Navickis RJ. A systematic review of the comparative safety of colloids. *Archives of Surgery* 2004; **139**(5): 552–63.

Cochrane Injuries Group Albumin Reviewers. Human albumin administration in critically ill patients: systematic review of randomised controlled trials. *British Medical Journal* 1998; **317**(7153): 235–40.

Finfer S, Bellomo R, Boyce N, French J, Myburgh J, Norton R. A comparison of albumin and saline for fluid resuscitation in the intensive care unit. *New England Journal of Medicine* 2004; **350**(22): 2247–56.

Maitland K, Pamba A, English M, Peshu N, Marsh K, Newton C, Levin M. Randomized trial of volume expansion with albumin or saline in children with severe malaria: preliminary evidence of albumin benefit. *Clinical Infectious Diseases* 2005; **40**(4): 538–45.

Schierhout G, Roberts I. Fluid resuscitation with colloid or crystalloid solutions in critically ill patients: a systematic review of randomised trials. *British Medical Journal* 1998; **316**(7136): 961–4.

Schortgen F, Lacherade JC, Bruneel F, Cattaneo I, Hemery F, Lemaire F, Brochard L. Effects of hydroxyethylstarch and gelatin on renal function in severe sepsis: a multicentre randomised study. *Lancet* 2001; **357**(9260): 911–16.

Velanovich V. Crystalloid versus colloid fluid resuscitation: a meta-analysis of mortality. *Surgery* 1989; **105**(1): 65–71.

Vercueil A, Grocott MPW, Mythen MG. Physiology, pharmacology, and rationale for colloid administration for the maintenance of effective hemodynamic stability in critically ill patients. *Transfusion Medicine Reviews* 2005; **19**(2): 93–109.

CHAPTER 10

Treatment of Massive Haemorrhage in Surgery and Trauma

Tim Walsh

OVERVIEW

- Immediate management of massive haemorrhage should focus on the ABC resuscitation principles. All patients should receive supplemental oxygen, two large-bore cannulae, samples taken for haematology, coagulation, biochemistry and blood grouping, and administration of intravenous fluid.

- Controlling the source of bleeding is a priority. Until there is source control, moderate hypotension (mean arterial pressure of 60–70 mmHg) is safe and preferable to hypervolaemia and/or normotension.

- Blood transfusion is life saving in massive haemorrhage, but it is important to remember that the haemoglobin concentration is influenced by plasma volume.

- All hospitals should have a major haemorrhage protocol to coordinate the clinical and laboratory response.

- After initial stabilization, the aim is to prevent or reverse complications that worsen outcomes such as hypothermia, electrolyte disturbances, metabolic acidosis and coagulopathy. This can be achieved through close monitoring, including near-patient techniques.

The normal circulating blood volume is 70–80 ml/kg body weight or approximately 5 L for a 70 kg adult. There is no universally agreed definition of massive haemorrhage, but the replacement of the patient's entire blood volume in <24 hours is commonly used. Significant acute blood loss rapidly results in hypovolaemic shock unless managed appropriately.

Untreated haemorrhagic shock can result in rapid death due to ischaemia of the organs. After treatment is initiated, further complications can arise as a result of deficiencies in blood clotting, hypothermia or electrolyte and acid–base imbalance. It is useful to broadly consider aspects of treatment in two phases: (i) the initial resuscitation phase; and (ii) later complications of resuscitation.

ABC of Transfusion, 4th edition, 2009. Edited by Marcela Contreras. © 2009 Blackwell Publishing, ISBN: 978-1-4051-5646-2.

Initial resuscitation phase

Physiological responses to haemorrhage

Acute haemorrhage results in the loss of circulating blood volume, which initiates reflex compensatory mechanisms to maintain organ perfusion. These principally involve activation of the sympathetic nervous system to constrict venous beds in the gut (splanchnic circulation) and skin. This vasoconstriction reduces the capacity of the circulation to increase venous return to the heart, which helps maintain the cardiac output. Cardiac output is also enhanced by a direct effect of sympathetic nerves on the atrial node, and increased circulating adrenaline, which act to increase the heart rate and contractility. Sympathetic system activation also constricts the arterioles via the sympathetic nerves, increasing the overall resistance of the circulation (increased cardiac afterload). The net result is the maintenance of a blood pressure sufficient to perfuse vital organs, principally the heart, brain and kidneys. The heart is particularly at risk during massive haemorrhage because its blood supply via the coronary arteries occurs only during diastole, when it normally extracts most of the available oxygen from haemoglobin (the oxygen extraction ratio is 60–70% compared to 20–40% in most other organs). If the oxygen supply to the heart is inadequate, death will rapidly follow.

Assessing the extent of haemorrhage

Clinical signs

Key early signs of significant haemorrhage are tachycardia and pallor (due to vasoconstriction in the skin). Hypotension, cardiac ischaemia, altered consciousness level and oliguria indicate that compensatory physiological mechanisms are not maintaining normal vital organ perfusion and are signs of severe haemorrhage. A commonly used classification relating the percentage blood loss to typical associated clinical signs is shown in Table 10.1.

Measured blood loss

In the emergency setting, particularly outwith the operating theatre, accurate measurements of blood loss are difficult. Visible blood loss is often overestimated and non-visible blood loss, for example retroperitoneal or around major bones, is difficult to quantify. In the operating theatre, ongoing blood loss should be monitored by weighing swabs, and recording the losses in suction or drain

Table 10.1 A commonly used classification of hypovolaemic shock (Baskett's classification).

	Class I	Class II	Class III	Class IV
Blood loss				
Percentage of .blood	<15	15–30	30–40	>40
Volume of blood (in 70 kg male) (L)	750	800–1500	1500–2000	>2000
Blood pressure				
Systolic	Unchanged	Normal	Reduced	Very low
Diastolic	Unchanged	Raised (narrowed pulse pressure)	Reduced	Very low
Pulse rate	Mild tachycardia	100–120	>120 (reduced volume)	>120 (very weak)
Capillary refill	Normal	Slow (>2 s)	Slow (>2 s)	Undetectable
Respiratory rate	Normal	Normal	Tachypnoea (>20/min)	Tachypnoea (>20/min)
Urine flow rate (ml/h)	>30	20–30	10–20	0–10
Extremities	Normal colour	Pale	Pale	Pale and cold
Complexion	Normal	Pale	Pale	Ashen
Mental state	Alert	Anxious and/or aggressive	Anxious and/or aggressive and/or drowsy	Drowsy and/or confused or unconscious

bottles. These measures are often inaccurate and should be used in conjunction with clinical signs.

Factors modifying normal physiological responses to haemorrhage

Concurrent medication is the commonest reason for non-typical physiological responses to haemorrhage. Tachycardia is unreliable in patients taking β-blocker drugs or other drugs that can slow the heart rate. This can result in an underestimation of blood loss severity. Patients on vasodilator drugs may have an exaggerated hypotensive response, for example angiotensin-converting enzyme (ACE) inhibitors or calcium channel blockers.

Initial investigations and procedures

In the emergency setting, the patient should be managed using the ABC resuscitation principles. Two large-bore cannulae should be established and samples taken for haematology, coagulation, biochemistry and blood grouping. Requests for immediate laboratory processing should be made.

All hospitals should have an agreed protocol that can be triggered in the event of major haemorrhage. An example is shown in Figure 10.1. Key elements include:

- a reliable mechanism for transporting samples and blood components to the laboratories and to the patient
- a predetermined 'pack' of blood components to avoid confusion or delays
- a mechanism to alert relevant individuals such as blood bank staff, haematologists and porters.

Principles of treatment

Oxygen therapy

High flow oxygen therapy, preferably using a rebreathing mask that enables the delivery of inspired oxygen >60%, should always be administered. This ensures maximum saturation of available haemoglobin, increases dissolved plasma oxygen, and induces some constriction of blood vessels (hyperoxic vasoconstriction) that may help maintain blood pressure.

Fluid therapy

Initial fluid resuscitation aims to restore an adequate circulating volume. This is usually judged best by improvement in blood pressure, falling heart rate, better capillary return and peripheral temperature. In severe cases, signs of better organ perfusion such as improving conscious level are useful guides.

The choice of fluid therapy is much debated. The most important principle is to relate the estimated expansion in circulating volume required to the predicted volume expected to remain in the circulation after redistribution. Initial resuscitation with approximately 20 ml/kg body weight of a crystalloid solution (1–2 L for a 70 kg adult) is appropriate for most clinical situations. During this period the degree of haemorrhage can be assessed from the history, clinical signs and response to fluid therapy. The options for subsequent fluids include a combination of:

- further crystalloids
- colloid solutions
- red cells
- coagulation factors.

The relevant properties of each fluid type, which are useful to consider in decision-making, are shown in Table 10.2. In practice, the combination administered will depend on the clinical condition of the patient, the results of blood tests and clinical judgment.

Source of bleeding control

Following initial resuscitation, the priority is to identify the source of bleeding and control it. This may require urgent transfer to the operating theatre or other specialist department depending on the site of haemorrhage. Delays to achieving source control can adversely affect patient outcome, especially when the haemorrhage is ongoing.

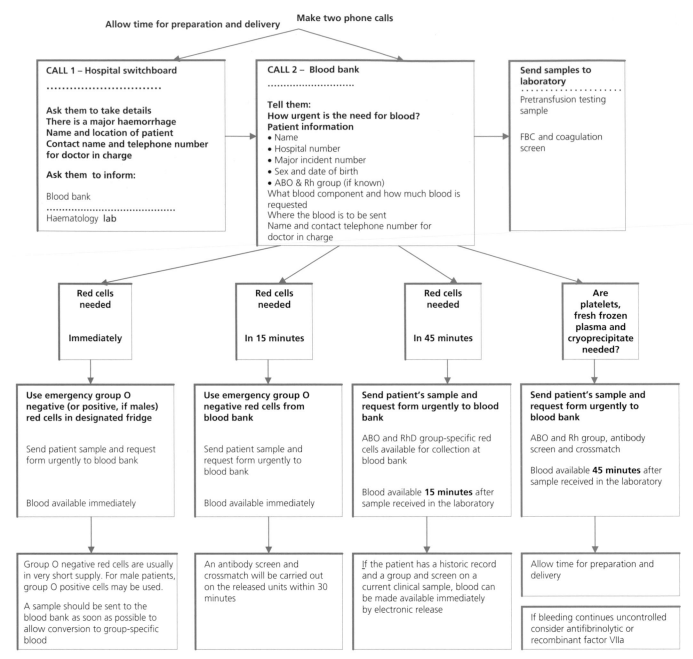

Figure 10.1 An example of a major haemorrhage protocol.

Target blood pressure prior to source control

Considerable research as been undertaken to determine the optimum blood pressure during resuscitation from massive haemorrhage, especially following major trauma. Current evidence supports partial correction of blood pressure to mean arterial pressure values of 60–70 mmHg, using incremental fluid therapy, until the source of bleeding is controlled. The lower blood pressure reduces blood loss from damaged vessels and increases the chance of stable clot formation. After source control, more aggressive restoration of normal blood pressure with fluids is appropriate to preserve organ function.

Optimum haemoglobin during massive haemorrhage

During haemorrhage, the haemoglobin concentration is strongly influenced by the plasma volume. Resuscitation with crystalloid and colloid fluids increases plasma volume. As a result, haemoglobin values can be misleadingly high prior to resuscitation and can decrease rapidly during fluid therapy. Measured haemoglobin concentrations need to be interpreted in the context of the time when sampling occurred, because they may correlate poorly with the circulating red cell mass (Figure 10.2). When the patient is unstable, the estimated blood loss together with clinical signs are the best guide to when red cells should be transfused. The choice of

Table 10.2 Important properties of intravenous fluids.

Fluid type	Volume of 1000 ml infusion remaining in circulation after distribution	Tonicity	Na+ and Cl− concentrations (mmol/L)	pH	Comments
5% dextrose	60–80 ml	Hypotonic	Na+: 0 Cl−: 0	4.0	No value as a resuscitation fluid
Normal (0.9%) saline	200–250 ml	Isotonic	Na+: 154 Cl−: 154	5.0	Excessive administration can contribute to acidosis (hyperchloraemic acidosis)
Ringer's lactate	200–250 ml	Isotonic	Na+: 131 Cl−: 112	6.5	Less likely to contribute to acidosis after initial resuscitation, but contains potassium and lactate, so caution in early phase
Haemaccel (succinylated gelatin)	1000 ml	Isotonic	Na+: 145 Cl−: 145	7.4	Half-life in circulation depends on rate of metabolism of colloid particles; it is typically 4 h
Gelofusine (polygeline gelatin)	1000 ml	Isotonic	Na+: 154 Cl−: 125	7.4	Half-life in circulation depends on rate of metabolism of colloid particles; it is typically 5 h
Hetastarch (example of starch solution-several available)	1000 ml	Isotonic	Na+: 154 Cl−: 154	5.5	Various starch solutions are available. Their exact properties depend on the specific product. Some expand intravascular volume more than infusion volume through high oncotic pressure
Plasma protein fraction (human albumin solution 4.5%)	1000 ml	Isotonic	Na+: 150 Cl−: 120	7.4	Evidence indicates no benefit over cheaper, non-human derived fluids

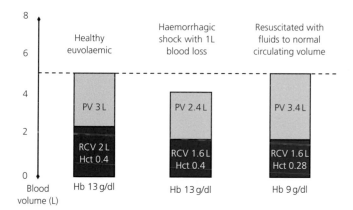

Figure 10.2 Relation between haemoglobin (Hb) concentration and plasma volume before and after resuscitation with fluids. Hct, haematocrit; RCV, red cell volume; PV, plasma volume.

red cell product should be determined by the perceived urgency of transfusion using clinical judgment (see Figure 10.1).

Once circulating volume has been restored, the haemoglobin concentration is a more reliable transfusion trigger. Although humans can tolerate haemoglobin concentrations of 4–5 g/dl under controlled conditions, these are not considered safe in clinical practice. A haemoglobin value of 7–9 g/dl is supported by available randomized trials in non-bleeding, critically ill patients. A value of 8–10 g/dl offers a 'safety margin' for further bleeding. Patients with heart disease should be kept at the upper end of this range.

Patient monitoring

As soon as available, patients should have continuous pulse oximetry, electrocardiogram and frequent non-invasive blood pressure

monitoring, in addition to the measurement of body temperature and respiratory rate. Invasive cardiovascular monitoring using arterial and central venous catheters are valuable, particularly during ongoing treatment. Placement of these catheters is often technically difficult in shocked patients, and should not be undertaken by inexperienced staff. Attempts should not distract clinicians from resuscitation.

Later complications of massive haemorrhage

Coagulopathy

Coagulopathy is an important component of the vicious circle that characterizes loss of control of the clinical condition. It is often multifactorial. Management relies on detection and correction of the contributing factors:

1 *Dilution of coagulation factors* in plasma occurs following massive transfusion. Protocolized prescriptions of blood components according to predicted blood loss or red cell transfusions are not recommended. Coagulation factor deficiency is likely after the loss of 1–1.5 blood volumes. Blood component administration should be guided by clinical evaluation (oozing or failure to generate clot) together with coagulation tests (see below).

2 *Thrombocytopenia* can occur due to dilution and consumption. Platelets usually remain at a level >50 × 10^9/L until >1.5 blood volumes have been replaced.

3 *Hypothermia* is a common and serious complication because it has multiple adverse effects (Table 10.3). Hypothermia can be prevented by using fluid warming devices (Figure 10.3) capable of rapidly warming infused fluids to body temperature. Modern patient warming devices are also highly efficient.

Table 10.3 Some adverse effects of hypothermia.

- Reduction in cellular enzyme activity and membrane pumps
- Reduction in cellular energy production (ATP); increased anaerobic metabolism and lactic acidosis
- Vasoconstriction and worsening organ perfusion
- Altered drug metabolism
- Impaired cardiac function and increased risk of arrythmias
- Impaired platelet function
- Coagulopathy due to altered coagulation enzyme activity and coagulation factor production
- Reduced immune function and susceptibility to infection

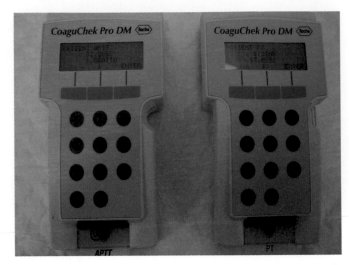

Figure 10.4 Devices that can measure prothrombin time (PT) and activated partial thromboplastin time (APTT) at the bedside.

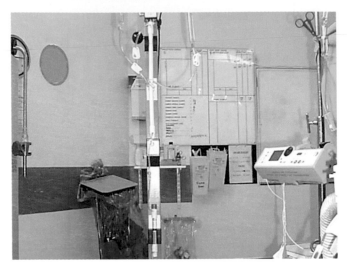

Figure 10.3 A blood and fluid warming device, capable of warming fluids from 4°C to body temperature even at high infusion rates.

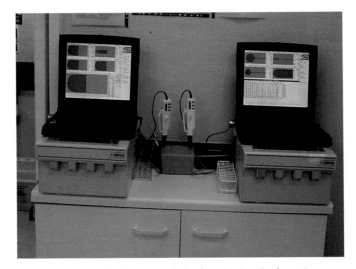

Figure 10.5 A thromboelastogram device for analyzing clot formation near the patient.

4 *Acidosis* is associated with adverse outcomes. Most blood gas analysers now measure pH and lactate; trends in both are useful guides to the effectiveness of ongoing resuscitation. Treatment relies on source control, effective resuscitation and prevention of hypothermia. Treatment with intravenous bicarbonate is rarely indicated.

5 *Hyperkalaemia* usually results from large transfusions with stored red cells, in which potassium leaks from erythrocytes. Acidosis and renal failure are other contributing factors. Treatment using standard protocols is recommended, but once transfused red cells recover and take up potassium it is not uncommon for supplementation to be required later.

6 *Hypocalcaemia* is relatively rare with modern blood components, but mainly results from citrate, which is highest in platelets. Routine calcium replacement is not recommended. Many blood analyzers measure ionized calcium, which is a better guide than total calcium. Low calcium can be corrected with intravenous calcium chloride or gluconate by slow infusion. Hypothermia and liver disease increase the risk of hypocalcaemia.

Monitoring coagulation

Regular laboratory coagulation testing to detect platelet and factor deficiencies (prothrombin time ratio (PTR), activated partial thromboplastin time ratio (APPTR), fibrinogen concentration) should be carried out in collaboration with a haematologist. Some of these tests can also be performed using automated kits at the bedside (Figure 10.4). During major haemorrhage, laboratory coagulation testing is advisable: (i) after approximately every 30–50% blood volume replacement; (ii) after infusion of blood components; or (iii) every 4 hours.

Thromboelastography is becoming established as a rapid method for assessing coagulation abnormalities. It can be performed near the patient using commercially available devices (Figure 10.5). Clot formation is analyzed dynamically by measuring the forces developed over time between the edges of a small cup, in which patient blood is placed, and a rod lowered into the blood sample. Various substances can be added to the cup to accelerate the start of clot formation or to evaluate specific aspects of clot formation, such as aprotinin (to abolish fibrinolysis) or heparinase (to reverse heparin effects) (Figure 10.6). Characteristic changes in the shape of the

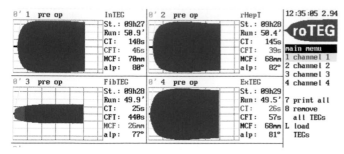

Figure 10.6 A thromboelastogram trace from a patient prior to major vascular surgery. Each channel is a different assessment of clot formation created by adding different substances to the sample to inhibit aspects of coagulation.

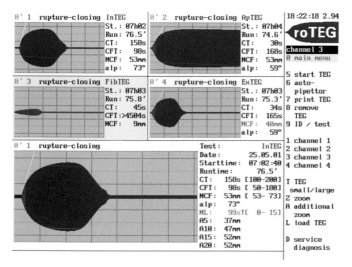

Figure 10.7 An abnormal thromboelastogram trace from a patient with severe coagulopathy from massive haemorrhage. The characteristic 'onion' shape of the trace indicates fibrinolysis. The top right panel is relatively normal because aprotinin was added to the sample, showing that this drug would be an effective treatment for the patient.

trace can guide the use of blood components and drugs to correct coagulopathy (Figure 10.7).

Treatment of coagulopathy

Coagulation factors

The PTR and APPTR should be kept at <1.5 by using fresh frozen plasma. Recommended dosing is 15 ml/kg (3–4 units for adults) per dose, although higher doses may be required for complete correction. Fibrinogen concentration should be kept >1.0 g/L using fresh frozen plasma and/or cryoprecipitate. Platelet counts should be kept >50 × 10^9/L during ongoing haemorrhage. Using a transfusion trigger of 75 × 10^9/L is advisable if delays in delivery are anticipated.

Fibrinolysis

Fibrinolysis results from the activation of plasminogen to plasmin. It is more common with larger blood loss, when treatment is delayed, with extensive tissue damage and in the presence of acidosis

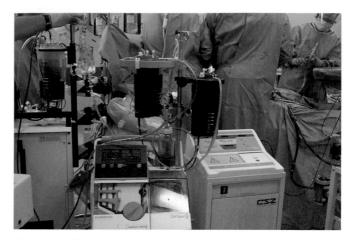

Figure 10.8 Effective use of cell salvage during surgery associated with major bleeding. The machine can recycle blood continuously during overwhelming blood loss, as in this case.

and hypothermia. It can be detected by measuring D-dimers (or an equivalent test) and from thromboelastography. Fibrinolysis can be treated with agents such as tranexamic acid in consultation with a haematologist. These drugs are sometimes used prophylactically for surgical procedures with a high risk of massive haemorrhage, such as complex cardiac surgery and liver transplantation. Recent evidence suggests that aprotinin may worsen long term outcomes in cardiac surgery patients and tranexamic acid appears a safer alternative.

Recombinant activated factor VII

This drug is not licensed for treatment of massive haemorrhage, but is increasingly used in this setting. Case reports and registries, and ongoing clinical trials, suggest a potential role in some patients. The drug promotes a 'thrombin burst', which may promote haemostasis when conventional measures have failed. It should only be used in consultation with a haematologist.

Recycling of autologous blood

Cell salvage and reinfusion of the patient's own blood is preferable to massive transfusion with allogeneic blood, which has undergone changes during storage that decrease the oxygen transport effectiveness of the red cells. Modern cell salvage devices can often be used during emergency situations, such as aortic aneurysm rupture and hepatic trauma (Figure 10.8; see Chapter 16).

Survival from major haemorrhage

Survival is increased by early intervention to control the source of bleeding and to prevent tissue ischaemia and organ failure. It is particularly important to avoid the combination of hypothermia, acidosis and coagulopathy (especially disseminated intravascular coagulation), which are associated with a high mortality.

Acknowledgments

The author thanks Dr Alastair Nimmo for providing the clinical pictures for this article.

Further reading

British Committee for Standards in Haematology. Guidelines on the management of massive blood loss. *British Journal of Haematology* 2006; **135**: 634–41.

Kwan I, Bunn F, Roberts I. Timing and volume of fluid administration for patients with bleeding. *Cochrane Database of Systematic Reviews* 2003, Issue 1. Art. No. CD002245.

Levi M, Peters M, Buller HR. Efficacy and safety of recombinant factor VIIa for treatment of severe bleeding: a systematic review. *Critical Care Medicine* 2005; **33**(4): 883–90.

McClelland DBL. *Handbook of Transfusion Medicine*, 4th edn. HM Stationery Office, London, 2007.

Spahn DR, Cerny V, Coats TJ. et al. Task Force for Advanced Bleeding Care in Trauma. Management of bleeding following major trauma: a European guideline. *Critical Care* 2007; **11**(1): R17.

CHAPTER 11

Immunological Complications of Blood Transfusion

Marcela Contreras and Cristina Navarrete

OVERVIEW

- Immunological complications of transfusion can be due either to: (i) antigens present in the transfused donor's cells or plasma reacting with the recipient's antibodies; or (ii) antibodies or lymphocytes present in the transfused donor's plasma reacting with antigens or cells in the recipient.

- The most frequent serious complications of transfusion are acute haemolytic transfusion reactions due to ABO blood group incompatibility and transfusion-related acute lung injury (TRALI). ABO incompatibility is caused by giving the wrong blood to a patient. TRALI is caused by white cell antibodies present in the donor's plasma reacting with incompatible cells in the recipient.

- Overall, the most frequent but not serious complications of transfusion are non-haemolytic febrile transfusion reactions and urticaria. The former have considerably decreased in the UK, since the introduction of universal leucodepletion.

Table 11.1 Immunological complications of blood transfusion.

		Percentage frequency
Red cells	Haemolytic reactions:	
	Immediate	0.02
	Delayed	0.2
White cells	Febrile reactions[*]	5.10
	Acute lung injury	<0.01
Platelets	Post-transfusion purpura	<0.01
Plasma proteins:		
Native	Anaphylaxis	<0.01
Ingested	Urticaria	1–3

[*] The incidence of febrile transfusion reactions has decreased significantly since the introduction of leucodepletion of red cells and platelets. It is now estimated to have a frequency of 0.1–0.2% or less.

The transfusion of blood or its components can correct many deficiencies, even if only temporarily, and in most cases this effect can be achieved without any untoward effects. Nevertheless, incompatibilities of several kinds do occasionally cause trouble. Each blood cell has many different antigens on its surface, so the cells of a donor are virtually certain to contain antigens different from those of the recipient. In addition, the donor's plasma may contain proteins that are foreign to the recipient. The donor's plasma may also contain antibodies incompatible with antigens carried by cells in the recipient (for example, transfusion of group O plasma to a group A patient). Fortunately the transfusion of blood cells or plasma containing foreign antigens causes an immediate reaction only when the recipient's serum contains a corresponding antibody, and then only rarely. In practice, severe reactions (caused, for example, by transfusion of incompatible red cells) are rare (Table 11.1), whereas mild reactions (caused, for example, by

reactions to foreign protein or hapten ingested by the donor and characterized by urticaria) are common.

Reactions to incompatible red cells

For a number of reasons, antibodies to red cell antigens are the most important in blood transfusion. Firstly, the volume of red cells transfused is usually greater than that of white cells or platelets, so that if incompatible red cells are transfused, the consequences are comparatively severe. Secondly, most individuals have 'naturally occurring' antibodies to either blood group A and/or B present on red cells. Thirdly, antibodies evoked by transfusions or pregnancy in women of childbearing age may subsequently cause haemolytic disease in their offspring.

Naturally occurring antibodies and immune antibodies to red blood cells

Some antibodies are found in subjects who have never been exposed to foreign blood cells, and the most important of these so-called 'naturally occurring' antibodies are anti-A, anti-B and

ABC of Transfusion, 4th edition, 2009. Edited by Marcela Contreras. © 2009 Blackwell Publishing, ISBN: 978-1-4051-5646-2.

Box 11.1 **Antibodies**

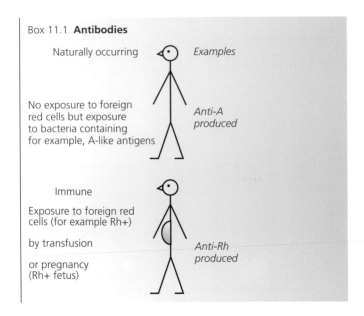

Box 11.2 **Haemolytic reactions**

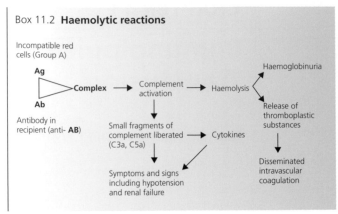

Box 11.3 **Immunological complications**

Incompatibility to:
- Red cells – Haemolysis:
  - intravascular (ABO)
  - extravascular (Rh)
- White cells
- Platelets
- Plasma proteins

Immune modulation:
- Beneficial
- Detrimental

Box 11.4 **Circumstances in which most incompatible transfusions are given**

Patient wrongly identified because:
- Unconscious (operation)
- Wristband removed during operation
- Human error
- Sample for pretransfusion tests taken from the wrong patient

anti-AB (Box 11.1). Most others are 'immune' antibodies and arise only after transfusion, or after pregnancy, when small numbers of fetal red cells enter the maternal circulation and may immunise the mother to antigens that the fetus has inherited from the father (see Chapter 6). Anti-RhD is the most common (and clinically significant) immune antibody against red blood cells.

Most incompatible transfusions are caused not by serological errors but by giving blood to the 'wrong' patient, that is, to a different patient from the one whose serum was tested before transfusion. The frequency with which incompatible transfusions are given is unknown, but their incidence is underreported; published estimates range from about 1/1000 to 1/20 000 transfusions (see Chapter 15).

Immediate haemolytic transfusion reactions

An immediate haemolytic transfusion reaction means the occurrence of signs of increased destruction of red cells soon after a transfusion. Mild haemolytic reactions may be caused in various ways – for example by transfusing blood that has been stored for too long – but severe haemolytic reactions are almost always caused by transfusing incompatible red cells (in most cases ABO incompatible) (Boxes 11.2 and 11.3).

Potent ABO antibodies present in group O plasma (usually in the form of fresh frozen plasma or platelets, but also in whole blood and, in the past, some fractionated blood products) may lead to severe haemolysis in group A, B or AB recipients. The following are the main reasons why ABO incompatibility plays such a large part:

1 Anti-A, anti-B and anti-AB are the most common blood group antibodies. They are present in the plasma of all subjects whose red cells lack the corresponding antigens. For example, a person of group O always has anti-A, anti-B and anti-AB in the plasma.
2 If a mistake is made in identifying a patient and the wrong blood is transfused (that is, blood that has been selected for a different patient), the chance (in a white subject) that it will be ABO incompatible is as high as one in three.

3 Anti-A and anti-B are usually potent immunoglobulin M (IgM) antibodies (especially in group O subjects) and by activating the full complement pathway produce rapid intravascular lysis of incompatible red cells so that, if reactions to ABO incompatible blood occur, they are usually severe. Fortunately, the resulting morbidity is of the order of 20% and mortality is less than 10%.

The following features of haemolytic transfusion reactions are the result of transfusion of ABO incompatible red cells.

Circumstances

As the cause of most incompatible transfusions is failure to identify the recipient correctly, many of such transfusions are given in emergencies and in surroundings where patients are not well known to those who are attending to them (Box 11.4). Thus most are given in operating theatres or intensive care units. Some patients who receive

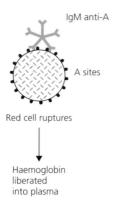

Figure 11.1 IgM anti-A binding to two adjacent A sites activates the whole of complement pathway (C1 to C9); C8 and C9 make holes in the red cell membrane.

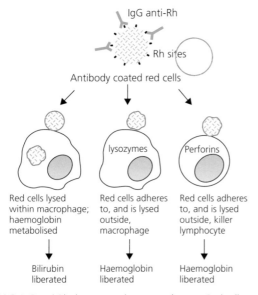

Figure 11.2 IgG anti-Rh does not activate complement. Red cells coated with antibody adhere to a macrophage or killer lymphocyte and are either ingested or lysed at the cell surface.

incompatible blood are unconscious at the time, so that there are no symptoms that might call attention to what is happening.

Mechanisms of red cell destruction

When ABO incompatible red cells are transfused – for example donor group A and recipient group O – the incompatible IgM antibody (anti-A and anti-AB in this case) immediately binds to the donor's red cells (Figure 11.1). The bound antibody activates complement leading to immediate lysis of donor red cells in the plasma. When the antibody is potent, virtually all the transfused red cells may be lysed within the bloodstream. Many other blood group alloantibodies, leading to immediate haemolytic reactions, are IgG and activate complement, but as a rule they do so only partially, up to C3b, and the coated cells, after binding to monocytes/macrophages, are either ingested or destroyed by cytotoxicity as they pass through the liver and spleen. Some antibodies – for example anti-Rh and a few anti-human leucocyte antigen (anti-HLA) – do not activate

Table 11.2 Immune red cell destruction.

Site of destruction	Predominantly intravascular	Predominantly extravascular
Characteristics of antibodies	Potent, lytic	Antibodies that do not activate or only partially activate complement
	(Anti-A and -B)	(Anti-Rh, anti-K, anti-Jk, and others)
Symptoms	Substernal pain, lumbar pain, restlessness	Nausea, shivering
Signs:		
Immediate	Hypotension, fever, uncontrollable bleeding	Fever
Later	Haemoglobinuria	Jaundice

complement (Figure 11.2), and these cause macrophages to remove coated red cells or platelets in the spleen only.

Symptoms and signs

The vast majority of patients experiencing an ABO incompatible transfusion reaction have no symptoms. However, about 20–25% of patients, particularly if group O, will have symptoms of varying severity (Table 11.2). In the conscious patient, the transfusion of even a few millilitres of ABO incompatible blood may cause symptoms within 1 or 2 minutes. The patient becomes restless and complains of a feeling of oppression that is often accompanied by substernal pain, chills and fever. The patient may also complain of a burning face and may have abdominal pain and may vomit. In the unconscious patient the most important signs are hypotension and uncontrollable bleeding.

The main cause of the symptoms and of the hypotension is the release of the products of complement (C3a and C5a) into the plasma. These are polypeptides with a molecular weight of about 20 000, which cause the contraction of smooth muscle and the production of nitric oxide, oxygen radicals and cytokines such as tumour necrosis factor (TNF) and interleukin-1 (IL-1); they also cause degranulation of mast cells leading to the release of vasoactive substances (bradykinin and serotonin). Bleeding is caused by disseminated intravascular coagulation, which is thought to be triggered by procoagulant substances released from red cell stroma after lysis and also, possibly, by the direct activation of the coagulation system by complement, by antigen–antibody complexes and by cytokines.

Oliguria is common after the transfusion of ABO incompatible blood and is thought to be the result of changes in renal blood flow precipitated by hypotension, rather than haemoglobinuria (Box 11.5).

As soon as it is suspected that incompatible blood has been transfused, the transfusion should be stopped, and an intravenous infusion of crystalloid solution should be started to maintain urinary output. Frusemide 80–200 mg should be given

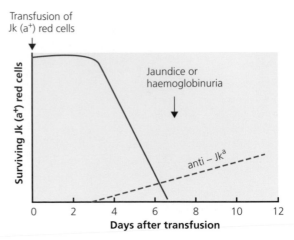

Figure 11.3 Delayed haemolytic transfusion reaction.

intravenously over 4 hours. The labels on the transfused unit and on all relevant blood samples should be checked and the laboratory notified; this is particularly important, because if the unit has been given to the wrong patient the right unit may have been – or may be about to be – given to another 'wrong' patient. If renal failure becomes established this can lead to death and the advice of a renal physician should be sought as soon as possible.

Although severe symptoms may follow the transfusion of only a few millilitres of incompatible red cells in group O patients with potent anti-A and anti-B, in patients with weak antibodies the transfusion of several units of ABO incompatible blood may cause only trivial effects. Very old and very young patients have weak ABO antibodies. As seen in Chapter 4, most recipients of blood in England belong to these age ranges.

Immediate haemolytic reactions as a result of transfusing incompatible red cells may also be caused by the presence of any other red cell antibodies active at 37°C in the recipient's blood. The next most common red cell antibody after anti-A and anti-B is anti-RhD. Rh antibodies are IgG, and extravascular haemolytic transfusion reactions caused by Rh incompatibility are usually much milder than those caused by ABO incompatibility. Other IgG antibodies, such as Kell, Duffy and Kidd, may also lead to extravascular haemolytic transfusion reactions. In Rh incompatibility fever is often the only sign of an adverse reaction, although jaundice, developing later, is quite common and, if IgG antibodies are very strong, haemoglobinuria caused by extravascular red cell destruction (not associated with renal failure) sometimes develops.

Delayed haemolytic transfusion reactions

These reactions occur in subjects who have been immunized to a foreign red cell antigen by an earlier transfusion or a previous pregnancy but in whom the concentration of antibody to the foreign antigen is so low that it cannot be detected by tests before the transfusion. Following the current transfusion of red cells containing the same foreign antigen there is a secondary immune response, and after a few days the concentration of IgG antibody has risen sufficiently to cause rapid destruction of those transfused red cells that contain the foreign antigen. The signs of a delayed haemolytic transfusion reaction are usually not noticed, but fever, a falling haemoglobin concentration and jaundice or, very rarely, haemoglobinuria, usually about 5–10 days after transfusion may occur (Figure 11.3). The specificities of the antibodies responsible for delayed haemolytic transfusion reactions are most often within the Rh system – that is, anti-c, anti-E and so on – or

Table 11.3 Antigens expressed on white blood cells and platelets.

	Class I (A,B,C)	HLA Class II (DR, DQ, DP)	HNA	HPA	ABO
Lymphocytes T	+	−*	−	−	−
Lymphocytes B	+	+	−	−	−
Monocytes	+	+	−	−	−
Granulocytes	+	−*	+	−	−
Dendritic cells	+	++	−	−	−
Platelets	+	−	−	+	+
Rbcs	+ᵃ	−	−	−	+
Plasma (soluble)	+	+	+	+	+

*On activated cells.
ᵃImmature rbc.

in the Kidd (Jk) system, but they may have other specificities such as anti-K.

Delayed haemolytic transfusion reactions occur after about one in 500 transfusions; alone they are seldom fatal, but they may have a serious adverse effect on a patient who is already gravely ill.

Reactions to incompatible white cells

White cells present in transfused products also express antigens which, if not identical to those present in the recipient, can be recognized as foreign (non-self) resulting in the development of antibodies responsible for some of the serious complications of blood transfusion. On the other hand, antibodies (and sometimes immune cells) present in the transfused product may react directly with the relevant antigens in the recipient and in this way provoke a transfusion reaction. The most important white cell antibodies are those reacting with HLA antigens present on all white cells and with the human neutrophil antigens (HNAs) found primarily on neutrophils. (See Table 11.3 for the expression of antigens on blood cells and plasma.)

In contrast to red cell antibodies, the majority of HLA (and up to a certain extent HNA) antibodies are of immune origin, i.e. they develop after exposure to foreign HLA or HNA molecules through pregnancy, transfusions or transplantation.

During pregnancy, the mother develops antibodies against the paternal HLA (as well as HNA and human platelet antigens (HPA)) specific antigens present in the fetus. These antibodies are normally IgG and of high affinity. Antibodies that develop following transfusions are a mixture of IgG and IgM, are often transient and can be detected in ~10% of previously transfused patients and in about 30–70% of multitransfused patients. Antibodies that develop following transplantation are predominantly IgG, but IgM can also be found transiently.

White cell antibodies present in blood transfusion recipients are implicated in the development of non-haemolytic febrile transfusion reactions (NHFTRs) and antibodies present in the transfused blood or blood component are associated with the development of transfusion-related acute lung injury (TRALI). On the other hand, viable lymphocytes present in blood or blood components are responsible for the development of transfusion-associated graft-versus-host disease (TA-GvHD).

Non-haemolytic febrile transfusion reactions

In patients whose plasma contains potent leucocyte antibodies (mostly HLA but also HNA and sometimes platelet-specific antibodies), the transfusion of whole blood or blood components containing incompatible leucocytes or platelets may provoke severe febrile reactions. The most common feature is fever, often preceded by shivering and beginning 30–60 minutes after the start of the transfusion. In some cases flushing of the face develops within 5 minutes of the start of the transfusion, presumably as a result of the release of cytokines and other pyrogens from the recipient's granulocytes and monocytes, stimulated by the products of complement activation or by activation of these cells when engulfing or lysing antibody-coated cells (Box 11.6).

Febrile reactions are quite common in patients who have previously been pregnant or who have had transfusions that have stimulated the formation of leucocyte antibodies. Most reactions are mild and can be dealt with by slowing the transfusion and giving antipyretics. In patients who have had at least two severe febrile reactions, blood or platelets with a reduced white cell load or that are leucodepleted should be transfused – that is, blood that has either had the buffy coat removed or has been passed through a special leucodepletion filter. In most cases, the removal of buffy coats, which reduces the white cell content 10-fold, will be sufficient to avoid NHFTRs.

With the introduction of universal leucodepletion in the UK, NHFTRs have decreased significantly. However some mild febrile reactions remain, presumably caused by cytokines and other biological response modifiers such as TNFα, IL-1a, IL-6 or IL-8 released by the remaining leucocytes present in stored blood or platelet concentrates.

Transfusion-related acute lung injury

If the donor's plasma contains potent leucoagglutinins that are incompatible with the recipient's granulocytes, transfusion may cause a severe reaction characterized by chills, fever, a non-productive cough, dyspnoea and severe hypoxaemia occurring during or in the 6 hours after transfusion. A chest radiograph shows numerous bilateral pulmonary nodules – predominantly perihilar – with infiltration of the lower lung fields (Figure 11.4). Most cases require prompt mechanical ventilation. The donors are almost always multiparous women who have developed leucoagglutinins during pregnancy. This reaction is clinically indistinguishable from acute respiratory distress from other causes and there is no specific treatment, although symptoms usually improve within 48–96 hours with the pulmonary infiltrates receding within 1–4 days. These reactions occur in approximately one in 3000–5000 transfusions and 5–10% of cases are fatal. The main blood components involved are those containing large volumes of plasma such as fresh frozen plasma and platelets, but red blood cell concentrates have also been implicated. HLA class I and class II and HNA antibodies in donor plasma have been implicated in 80% of clinically convincing cases.

Box 11.6 **Febrile reaction to incompatible white cells**

Foreign leucocytes + leucocyte antibody

Destroyed by full complement activation

Engulfed by host monocytes

Release of pyrogen

FEVER

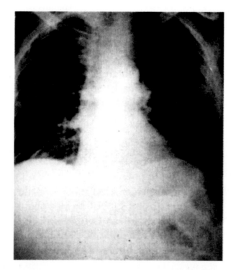

Figure 11.4 Chest radiograph of a patient who experienced a severe transfusion reaction as a result of potent leucoagglutinins in transfused plasma. There are numerous nodules, predominantly perihilar, and infiltration of the lower lung fields.

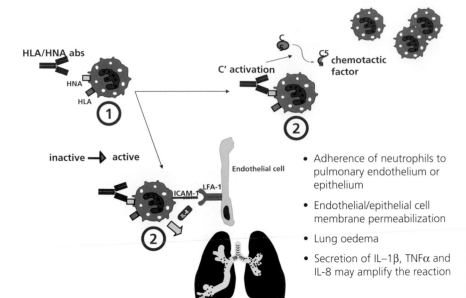

- Adherence of neutrophils to pulmonary endothelium or epithelium
- Endothelial/epithelial cell membrane permeabilization
- Lung oedema
- Secretion of IL–1β, TNFα and IL-8 may amplify the reaction

Figure 11.5 Diagram showing how TRALI occurs. HLA, human leucocyte antigen; HNA, human neutrophil antigen; ICAM-1, intercellular adhesion molecule; IL, interleukin; LFA-1, leucocyte function antigen; TNF, tumour necrosis factor.

These antibodies react with the leucocytes of the patient, triggering the activation of the neutrophils and the complement cascade, the release of chemotactic factors, sequestration of neutrophils in the small vessels of the lung, and ultimately damage to the vascular endothelium. There is an accumulation of leucocytes within the small vessels of the lung and lung oedema. Throughout this process there is secretion of inflammatory cytokines such as IL-1β and TNFα, which may induce and amplify the reaction (Figure 11.5).

Biologically active lipids present in stored, but not fresh, cellular blood components have been implicated by some, but other predisposing clinical conditions (e.g. recent surgery, cytokine therapy, active infection) also seem to be required. The laboratory investigations of these cases involve the screening of implicated donors for HLA and HNA antibodies. Female donors and male donors with a history of transfusion should be the first ones to be investigated and, if antibody positive, the patient should be typed for the relevant antigen. The gold standard test is a leucocyte crossmatch between the donor's plasma and the patient's white cells. A positive crossmatch confirms the diagnosis of TRALI.

Transfusion-associated graft-versus-host disease

This is a rare but usually fatal immunological complication of blood transfusion occurring approximately within 2 weeks of transfusion, which results from the engraftment and clonal expansion of viable, mostly HLA compatible, immunocompetent donor lymphocytes in an immunocompromised (though occasionally immunocompetent) host.

The clinical features classically include a skin rash, diarrhoea, fever, hepatitis and pancytopenia. Definitive diagnosis of TA-GvHD includes the detection of donor-derived cells or DNA in the blood or affected tissues of the recipient.

The incidence of TA-GvHD is not known, although it has been suggested that the disorder is underreported. The first 2 years of haemovigilance in the UK indicated that TA-GvHD was the most common recorded cause of transfusion-related death. The blood

Table 11.4 Leucocyte and platelet levels in blood.

Cell type	Blood count
Total leucocytes	$4.0–11.0 \times 10^9/L$
Neutrophils	$2.5–7.5 \times 10^9/L$
Eosinophils	$0.04–0.4 \times 10^9/L$
Basophils	$0.01–0.1 \times 10^9/L$
Monocytes	$0.2–0.8 \times 10^9/L$
Lymphocytes	$1.5–3.5 \times 10^9/L$
Platelets	$140–400 \times 10^9/L$

components implicated are those containing lymphoctyes and it can be prevented by the use of γ-irradiated blood components.

Reactions to incompatible platelets

Although it is doubtful whether platelets themselves can cause febrile reactions, transfusions of platelet concentrates quite often used to, because they contained contaminating leucocytes. In addition, because platelet concentrates contain plasma, all types of reactions due to plasma can be experienced by patients receiving platelet transfusions. (Table 11.4 details the usual ranges of leucocyte and platelet concentrations found in blood.)

Platelets can cause a serious kind of delayed reaction known as post-transfusion purpura, characterized by severe thrombocytopenia approximately 1 week post-transfusion (Figure 11.6). The patient has become sensitized to a foreign platelet antigen (most commonly HPA-1a, previously termed PI-Al), usually as a result of previous pregnancies but rarely by transfusion. After a later transfusion of blood with platelets carrying this antigen, a secondary response develops, and this leads to destruction of the patient's own HPA-1a negative platelets and severe thrombocytopenia. It is likely that the patient's own HPA-1a negative platelets are destroyed by autoantibodies produced as a result of

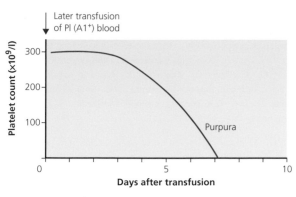

Figure 11.6 Post-transfusion purpura.

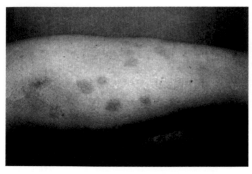

Figure 11.7 Urticaria is one of the commonest immunological complications of blood transfusion.

the original alloimmunization, which become stimulated with the second antigenic challenge.

Although the incidence of HPA-1a-negative subjects among Europeans is two in 100, post-transfusion purpura is rare and occurs in approximately one in 700 000 transfusions, usually in female patients. Onset is severe and sometimes fatal. The best treatment is large doses of immunoglobulin given intravenously or plasma exchange.

Immunological refractoriness to platelet transfusions

Platelet transfusion therapy plays a major role in the management of patients with haematological and oncological disorders with intermittent or long-lasting thrombocytopenia. However, some of these patients become refractory to the transfusion of platelets from random donors and this is characterized by the failure to gain adequate platelet count increments ($<10 \times 10^9$/l) 1 hour post transfusion. Platelet refractoriness may be the result of immunological and/or non-immunological causes. Immunological refractoriness, caused by antibody-mediated destruction of transfused platelets, is normally due to HLA antibodies, although antibodies against HPAs and high titre ABO antibodies have also been implicated occasionally.

Different approaches are currently being used for the management of immunological platelet refractoriness including: (i) the provision of crossmatch-compatible platelets; (ii) the use of platelets negative for the HLA antigen(s) corresponding to the patient's HLA antibody; and (iii) the use of complete or partially HLA-A and -B antigen-matched platelets from unrelated donors. All these different approaches have been shown to be effective. Although platelets express HLA-A, -B and -Cw antigens, matching at the HLA-A and -B locus antigens only is required.

The laboratory investigations to identify these cases and provide HLA-matched platelets include:
- screening for and detection of HLA-specific antibodies
- definition of antibody specificity
- HLA typing of patients
- selection and issue of HLA-compatible platelets from a large panel of HLA-typed platelet donors
- documentation of post-transfusion increments.

Reactions to plasma proteins

The commonest adverse reaction to plasma (or any blood component containing plasma) is urticaria (hives) (Figure 11.7). In fact, 1–3% of patients transfused with plasma experience urticaria. The cause is presumably a reaction between plasma proteins or some foreign allergen (for example from pollen or milk) present in the donor's plasma and a corresponding IgE antibody in the recipient. Urticaria is usually mild, but if it is severe it can be treated by slowing the transfusion and giving an antihistamine (e.g. chlorpheniramine 10 mg i.v. or i.m.). Patients who have developed urticaria after previous transfusions may be given antihistamine orally before subsequent transfusions.

Rarely, severe anaphylactic reactions occur, and they are characterized by hypotension and even shock, a feeling of a 'lump' in the throat, stridor, substernal pain, chest tightness, wheezing, dyspnoea and gastrointestinal symptoms including abdominal cramps. These signs and symptoms are usually the result of a reaction between normal IgA in the donor's plasma and so-called class-specific anti-IgA in the recipient's plasma. This antibody is found only in 'algA' subjects, who are almost completely deficient in IgA (<1 mg/L plasma). The incidence of algA subjects in the normal population is about one in 1000. However, severe anaphylactic reactions are extremely rare and can lead to death. They should be treated promptly by stopping the transfusion and giving adrenaline 0.5–1 mg subcutaneously or intramuscularly and hydrocortisone 100–200 mg intravenously. Anaphylactic reactions in patients with anti-IgA in their plasma can be prevented by using IgA-deficient donors or, if unavailable, well washed red cells.

Immunomodulatory effects of transfusion

Some, though not all, studies in humans and experimental animals argue in favour of an immunosuppressive effect of transfusion with a detrimental effect as regards to an increased rate of postoperative bacterial infection and an increased rate of recurrence of colorectal carcinoma. There is also a possible beneficial effect of some blood transfusions on the survival of renal allografts. It is not known which of the components of blood has a greater impact on the immune system, but leucocytes and especially lymphocytes are the favoured candidates.

Further reading

Bidwell J, Navarrete C, eds. *Histocompatibility Testing*. Imperial College Press, London, 2000.

Bax J. Transfusion-related acute lung injury (TRALI): a serious adverse event of transfusion. *Vox Sanguinis* 2005; **89**: 1–10.

Kleinman S. A perspective on transfusion-related acute lung injury two years after the Canadian Consensus Conference. *Transfusion* 2006; **46**: 1465–8.

Mollison PL, Engelfriet CP, Contreras M. *Blood Transfusion in Clinical Medicine*, 10th edn. Blackwell Scientific Publications, Oxford, 1997.

Navarrete C. The HLA system in blood transfusion. *Baillière's Clinical Haematology* 2000; **13**(4): 511–32.

CHAPTER 12

Infectious Complications of Blood Transfusion: Bacteria and Parasites

John Barbara and Marcela Contreras

OVERVIEW

- Careful selection of voluntary, unpaid donors remains a first key step to maximize blood safety.

- Although 'persistence' is the hallmark of transfusion infections, acute infections at high incidence may pose a threat.

- Bacterial infections are a major component of the residual microbial risks from transfusion in the developed world.

- Rigorous history taking is essential for reducing the risk of transmitting parasitic infections.

- Visual checks of the blood bag prior to transfusion should always be undertaken.

- Most countries screen blood donors for human immunodeficiency virus, hepatitis B and C virus and syphilis by appropriate donor selection and laboratory testing.

- Some countries also test for human T-cell leukaemia virus, cytomegalovirus, West Nile virus and Chagas' disease.

- Inactivation procedures have increased the safety of fractionated blood products and also of some labile blood components.

Box 12.1 **Ensuring a safe blood supply**

- Donor selection
- Microbiological screening tests
- Microbial inactivation

Box 12.2 **Screening tests for blood donations (see Chapter 1)**

Mandatory in the UK
- Hepatitis B surface antigen
- Antibody to human immunodeficiency virus 1 (HIV-1) and HIV-2 in combination with HIV antigen
- Antibody to *Treponema pallidum* (syphilis)
- Antibody to hepatitis C virus (HCV)
- Antibody to human T-cell leukaemia virus (HTLV) (on pooled samples)
- HCV genome detection or nucleic acid technology for HCV (on pooled samples)

Optional (for selected recipients)
- Antibody to cytomegalovirus

Optional (on selected donors with relevant history):
- Antibody to *Plasmodium falciparum* (malaria)
- Antibody to *Trypanosoma cruzi* (Chagas' disease)

Tests performed in some countries
- HIV genome detection
- Hepatitis B virus genome detection
- Antibody to hepatitis B core
- Alanine aminotransferase levels
- BI9 genome detection
- West Nile virus genome detection

Long before the transmission of human immunodeficiency virus (HIV) became a prominent potential hazard of blood transfusion, considerable expertise in preventing the transmission of infection by transfusion had already been developed in the blood services. The first and most important step in maintaining a safe blood supply will always be a rigorous process of selection of prospective voluntary, unpaid blood donors (Box 12.1; see Chapter 1). The second is the use of specific microbiological screening tests (Box 12.2). Agents transmissible by transfusion can be either cell associated – for example cytomegalovirus (CMV) and human T-cell leukaemia virus type 1 (HTLV-1) – or plasma associated – for example hepatitis B virus – or both (e.g. HIV). If they are plasma associated, pooling large numbers of units of plasma (e.g. 15 000–20 000 U as in the production of factor VIII) greatly increases the chances of disseminating such contaminants. Due to the separation of each unit of blood into its components, even

without pooling, transfusion of blood components may result in up to four or five patients being infected by a single contaminated donation. Fortunately, current inactivation procedures render fractionated plasma products virtually free of microbial infectivity. This offers a third approach to ensuring the transfusion of safe blood products and the concept is gradually being extended to labile components as well.

ABC of Transfusion, 4th edition, 2009. Edited by Marcela Contreras. © 2009 Blackwell Publishing, ISBN: 978-1-4051-5646-2.

Properties of infections transmissible by transfusion

Agents transmitted by blood transfusion often possess a combination of some or all of the following properties:

- they are present in the blood for long periods, sometimes in high titres
- they can cause subclinical infections or only mild symptoms
- they have long incubation periods (sometimes years) before clinical signs appear
- they may exist in a latent or carrier state, or both; they are stable in blood stored at 4°C.
- certain agents causing acute infection with only transient viraemia may be a threat if the rate of new (incident) infections is very high. An example is West Nile virus in North America.

Screening tests for blood donations

Screening tests are paradoxically usually directed at antibody to the agent rather than antigens from the agent, except in the case of hepatitis B virus. Antibody screening tests are markers for certain persistent or chronic infections and therefore indicate a potential for infectivity, especially when the inoculum is as large as a unit of blood or a blood component.

Various agents may be transmitted by transfusion, but in the UK there are only five serological screening tests for blood donations that are currently mandatory (Box 12.2). They are tests for: (i) hepatitis B surface antigen (HBsAg) for hepatitis B virus; (ii) antibody to HIV-1 and -2, in combination with HIV antigen; (iii) antibody to hepatitis C virus (HCV); (iv) antibody to *Treponema pallidum* (syphilis); and (v) antibody to HTLV performed on the pools of 48 samples used for detection of HCV genome (nucleic acid technology or NAT). Tests for several other agents are available, but it has not yet been considered necessary to extend the present range. The range of techniques for screening, to which process control can be applied, includes enzyme-linked immunosorbent assay (ELISA), haemagglutination and gelatin particle agglutination. For a test to be suitable for screening blood for transfusion, several conflicting demands have to be met.

Quality control of microbiological screening of blood donations for transfusion in the UK is essential because the occurrence of donations positive for hepatitis B virus, HIV, HCV or syphilis is rare. In contrast to blood grouping, in which every sample produces a 'positive' result of some sort, in microbiological screening tests most donor serum samples are negative. Great vigilance is therefore required in carrying out the routine screening tests (Figures 12.1 and 12.2). In low prevalence populations even an apparently low rate of false positive results from a screening test implies that a positive reaction has little predictive value. If, for example, an agent has an incidence of one in 100 000 donations, then a test with a specificity of 99.9% will produce a false positive reaction once in every 1000 donations, or 100 false positive reactions for every true positive (Table 12.1). It is therefore imperative that any donor samples that give a positive reaction in any of the mandatory screening tests should be sent to a reference laboratory for confirmation before the donor is informed of the results. Blood centres in the UK and

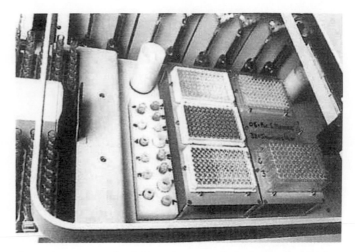

Figure 12.1 Reagents for ELISA can be automatically dispensed, with full process control.

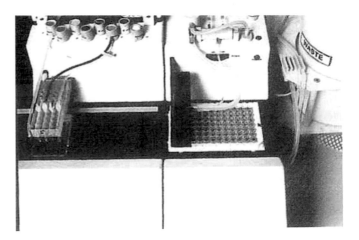

Figure 12.2 All assay steps can be performed automatically. Although microplate-based assays are illustrated here, fully enclosed systems such as the Abbot Laboratories PRISM™ machine are also in common use. This system has been fully assessed by the UK blood services to ensure that full process control of testing is achieved.

Table 12.1 Table of predictive values.

- Prevalence: 1 in 100 000
- Specificity: 99.9% (minimum UK requirement)
- False positive rate: 1 in 1000
- 100 false positives for every true positive

in other developed countries, use assays that have low false positive rates, and they all have access to centralized reference laboratories that carry out a battery of confirmatory tests, which virtually eliminates the possibility of mislabelling uninfected donors. In the UK these reference laboratories regularly coordinate their confirmation protocols.

Specificity of microbiological assays is vital if the confidence of donors is to be maintained, and it must not be forgotten in the search for increased sensitivity. Fortunately recombinant and synthetic antigens and modern molecular biological methods have produced remarkable improvements in the sensitivity and specificity of assays, such as those for detecting HIV infection.

Bacterial complications of transfusion

Bacteria comprising normal skin flora, such as staphylococci, can contaminate blood donations at the time of collection; the blood's own bactericidal powers, citrate and cold storage will, however, destroy many such contaminants. Due to their storage requirements at room temperature, platelet concentrates carry the highest risk of bacterial contamination.

Bacterial complications of transfusion are rare in the UK because of the use of sterile, disposable collection sets and clean phlebotomy techniques. When they do occur, however, they can rapidly be fatal, as a result of septicaemia, endotoxic shock, or both. Exogenous contaminants can be introduced into the blood mainly during collection or (rarely) during processing or the preparation and storage of platelets. At present, in the National Blood Service, all blood components are prepared in closed systems; blood is collected in multiple packs and the possibility of microbes entering the packs is negligible. Even washed red cells and frozen-thawed red cells are prepared in closed systems with the aid of sterile connecting devices. On the other hand, if any blood service prepares blood components in an open system, they should be processed in clean rooms and given a limited (24 hours) shelf life.

Serious and rarely fatal complications of blood transfusion may be caused by the accidental introduction of bacteria normally resident on the skin, such as staphylococci, diphtheroids and streptococci (Box 12.3). In addition, blood services across the world have also reported the rare accidental introduction of Gram-negative organisms, some of which were proven to also be present on the skin. To minimize the risk, in addition to rigorous arm cleansing (Figure 12.3), the first 20 ml of the donation which may contain the highest bacterial load is 'diverted' to a pouch and used to provide samples for laboratory testing. Other environmental contaminants

have also been reported as causing serious (and often fatal) bacterial infections; these include pseudomonads, *Achromobacter* spp. and unusual coliforms, some of which grow preferentially at 4–8°C or at room temperature, but not at 37°C. Such bacteria use citrate as a source of energy, and this leads to the clotting of stored blood.

Bacteria that may cause low grade or asymptomatic infections in the donor (such as *Salmonella* or *Yersinia* species) are sometimes an endogenous source of contamination. *Y. enterocolitica* can be a particular problem as it grows in red cell concentrates stored at 4°C without causing haemolysis and produces a powerful endotoxin.

Conversely, bacteria that do not grow in blood stored at 4°C may grow rapidly in platelet concentrates that are routinely stored for 5 days at 20–22°C. Contaminated platelet concentrates have been implicated in fatal episodes of *Salmonella* spp., *Escherichia coli* and staphylococcal septicaemia. All blood components should be visually inspected for evidence of bacterial contamination (e.g. as in Figure 12.4) prior to transfusion.

Reactions to the transfusion of contaminated blood result from the septicaemia itself, endotoxins, or both. They usually develop within minutes, with some or all of the following signs and symptoms: chills, rigors, fever, nausea, vomiting, bloody diarrhoea, abdominal and muscle pains, hypotension (often leading to shock with flushing and dry skin) or hypertension (rarely), with subsequent renal failure, haemoglobinuria and disseminated intravascular coagulation. It is very difficult to distinguish these symptoms from those caused by an ABO incompatible haemolytic transfusion reaction.

As soon as it is suspected that a contaminated unit is being – or has been – transfused, the transfusion should be stopped and blood samples as well as the packs of any units transfused should be sent to the blood bank and microbiology laboratory for investigation. The patient should be treated for shock before the results of laboratory investigations are available. Appropriate broad-spectrum antibiotics should be given intravenously, together with adequate fluid replacement and vasopressive drugs, as necessary.

Recently, the UK haemovigilance system, Serious Hazards of Transfusion (SHOT), had recorded some reduction in the number of bacterial transmissions. This may well be due to the implementation of diversion of the first 20 ml of blood collected and to enhanced arm cleansing. Continued monitoring is required to

---

Box 12.3 **Bacteria and parasites transmissible by blood transfusion**

Bacteria
- Occasional exogenous or endogenous bacterial contaminants (e.g. *Pseudomonas*, *Salmonella*)
- *Treponema pallidum* (syphilis)
- Brucellosis (donors giving a history are not accepted in the UK)

Parasites
- *Plasmodium* species (malaria)
- *Trypanosoma cruzi* (Chagas' disease): endemic in Latin America. The parasite is present in 75% of seropositive subjects. Between 1% and 22% of donors in Latin America are seropositive
- *Toxoplasma gondii*: only a risk in immunosuppressed patients transfused with granulocytes
- *Babesia microti* (Nantucket fever): potential risk in areas of North America
- *Leishmania donovanii*: occasional reports suggesting transmission

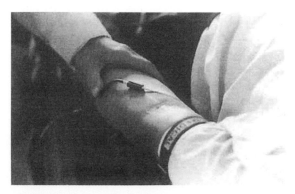

Figure 12.3 Taking a blood donation after thorough cleansing of the arm.

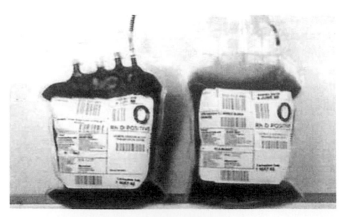

Figure 12.4 If units of blood are left to settle, bacterial haemolysis can be detected. Uninfected unit shows clear demarcation between the plasma and red cells (right), in contrast to a haemolysed unit (left).

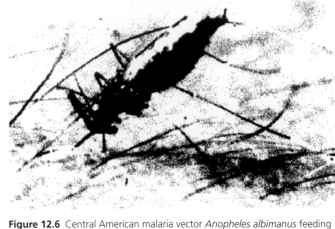

Figure 12.6 Central American malaria vector *Anopheles albimanus* feeding on a person. (Courtesy of Liverpool School of Tropical Medicine.)

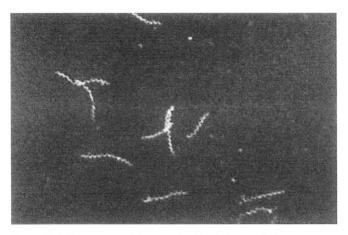

Figure 12.5 *Treponema pallidum* examined by dark ground microscopy (approximate length 7 µm). (Courtesy of Professor H.P. Lambert and Gower Medical Publishing.)

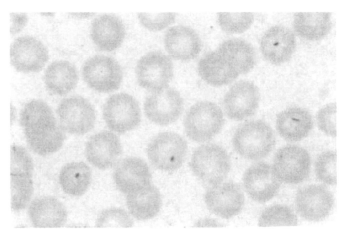

Figure 12.7 Ring forms of *Plasmodium falciparum* within red blood cells. (Courtesy of Dr P. Hewitt and Gower Medical Publishing.)

inform policy on the possible introduction of routine bacterial testing of platelet preparations as cases still occur.

Other complications of transfusion

Treponema pallidum (syphilis)

Treponema pallidum (Figure 12.5) can only be transmitted by fresh blood and platelet concentrates because it is readily inactivated by refrigeration for 72 hours. The incubation period varies from 4 weeks to 4.5 months, the average being 9–10 weeks. It is only rarely transmitted by transfusion, but when it is, it presents as a secondary eruption. It responds to treatment with antibiotics, usually a course of benzylpenicillin (2 megaunits).

Screening for the antibody is mandatory, in the UK, by specific *T. pallidum* haemagglutination or particle agglutination assays or ELISA. In early primary syphilis, at the height of infectivity, screening tests may be negative. The detection rate of infectious donors is low because most positive donors have had the infection and been treated. Donors with acute or latent infection, whilst

still relatively rare are now being seen more frequently. Screening for syphilis may also identify donors who have contracted other sexually transmitted diseases.

Malaria

Plasmodium falciparum is the most dangerous of the human malarial parasites; the others are *Plasmodium vivax*, *Plasmodium ovale* and *Plasmodium malariae*. They are transmitted between people by an insect vector (e.g. Figure 12.6). The organisms are absolutely restricted to red blood cells (Figure 12.7), which may also contaminate other blood components such as platelets. Freezing plasma will lyse any contaminated red cells and is therefore safe, but malaria parasites can survive storage of blood at 4°C for more than a week. The incubation period is from 1 week to 1 month, but for *P. malariae* it may be several months. Special note should be taken of unexplained fevers after transfusion.

Occasional transmissions still occur in the UK despite the careful taking of histories prior to donation. Of 18 374 cases of malaria in Britain reported to the Malaria Reference Laboratory between 1977 and 1986, only four were caused by blood transfusion. However, a case of fatal transfusion-transmitted malaria has subsequently been reported. Most countries exclude donors who may have been exposed to malarial infections on the basis of their clinical and travel history. In the UK a recently approved ELISA to detect antibody to *P. falciparum* has allowed the acceptance of donors with a history of possible malarial exposure provided that this exposure was more than 6 months previously and that they are seronegative and free of symptoms. If a diagnosis of malaria after transfusion is made, conventional treatment should be started. Primaquine should not be used, however, as in cases of transfusion-transmitted malaria the parasite will be restricted to the red cells.

Conclusion

Meticulous cleansing of the skin and a clean venepuncture technique are essential to reduce the risk of skin contaminants entering blood donations. Diversion of the first 20 ml of each blood donation appears to have reduced the number of bacterial transmissions. The following procedure should be carried out before all transfusions to minimize the chance of bacterial contamination:

1 Check that the pack is intact (no tears or pin holes).
2 Ensure that blood is stored at the correct temperature with minimal time spent at room temperature (except platelets).
3 Do not warm units of blood before transfusion.
4 Look at packs that have been standing undisturbed to see if there is evidence of haemolysis (for example a purple mass of red cells or brown red plasma) or clotting, which may be indicative of bacterial contamination The interface between cells and plasma should be clearly defined.

In order to minimize the risk of malarial transmission, history taking of donors should be rigorous.

Further reading

Barbara JAJ, Regan FAM, Contreras MC, eds. *Transfusion Microbiology.* Cambridge University Press, Cambridge, 2008.

Mollison PL, Engelfiet CP, Contreras M. Infectious agents transmitted by transfusion. In: *Blood Transfusion in Clinical Medicine*, 10th edn. Blackwell Science, Oxford, 1997, pp. 509–557.

Wendel S, Barbara JAJ. In: Lozano M, Contreras M, Blajchman M, eds. *Global Perspectives in Transfusion Medicine.* AABB Press, Bethesda, MD, 2006, pp. 55–101.

CHAPTER 13

Infectious Complications of Blood Transfusion: Viruses

John Barbara and Marcela Contreras

OVERVIEW

- In the absence of donor selection, self-exclusion and donation screening, many transfusion-transmitted infections are caused by viruses, mainly Hepatitis B and C viruses and HIV-1 and HIV-2.
- Nucleic acid detection (NAT) by genome amplification techniques is increasing in popularity.
- Incremental yields from NAT compared with antigen–antibody 'combi' assays relate to the incidence of infection and the length of the 'window period'.
- Pathogen inactivation/reduction of labile blood components has not yet achieved its full potential.
- National surveillance of complications of blood transfusion (haemovigilance) is a vital component of quality.
- See also overview for Chapter 12.

Many transfusion-transmitted infections are caused by viruses and continue to arouse considerable public and medical interest (Table 13.1). Effective antiviral agents are still not available to treat all viral infections, so the safety of blood and blood components relies on 'self-exclusion' by potential donors who are at risk of contracting viruses that are transmissible by transfusion (often transmitted sexually or by intravenous drug misuse) and on laboratory screening for evidence of microbial infection. So far, inactivation methods are only routinely used for fractionated products made from pooled plasma and for fresh frozen plasma (FFP). Photochemical methods to inactivate infectious agents and living cells in labile blood components have been developed. For example, psoralens together with ultraviolet light can irreversibly cross-link nucleic acids. Although a licensed commercial product is available for treating platelet preparations, it is not widely used. This chapter gives a brief review of the range of viruses that are transmitted by transfusion and of their properties.

Hepatitis B virus

The hepatitis B virus (HBV) is 42 nm in diameter and contains DNA (Figure 13.1). Reports of the isolation of cross-reacting

Table 13.1 Viruses transmissible by blood transfusion.

Plasma-borne viruses	Cell-associated viruses
Hepatitis A (rarely)	Cytomegalovirus
Hepatitis B and delta agent and Hepatitis B variants	Epstein–Barr virus (more than 95% of adults are immune)
Hepatitis C	Human herpes virus 8
Hepatitis E (rarely)	HTLV-1 (causes human T-cell leukaemia and tropical spastic paraparesis)
Other (non-hepatotropic) viruses (GBV-C/HGV; TTV; SEN-V)	HTLV-II (clinical relevance not clear; may be more common than HTLV-I in some countries)
HIV-1 and HIV-2 (also cellular)	HIV-1 and HIV-2 (also plasma borne)
Serum parvovirus B19	
West Nile virus	
Dengue virus	

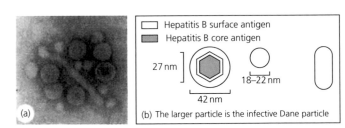

Figure 13.1 Hepatitis B virus particles: (a) electron micrograph, and (b) diagram. (Courtesy of Butterworth Scientific Ltd.)

variants of HBV have been published. The virus is plasma borne and easily transmitted by all blood components and most blood products (for example factor VIII). It is not transmitted by pasteurized albumin. The chance of transmission is enhanced when plasma is pooled for the manufacture of blood products. However, the risk is removed with current viral inactivation procedures of fractionated blood components. The incubation period ranges from 2 to 6 months but is usually about 4 months (Figure 13.2). Although it is extremely infectious parenterally and is resistant to both chemical and heat inactivation, the number of transfusion-transmitted cases has been drastically reduced by screening blood donations. The few cases that do occur are due to seronegative donors

ABC of Transfusion, 4th edition, 2009. Edited by Marcela Contreras. © 2009 Blackwell Publishing, ISBN: 978-1-4051-5646-2.

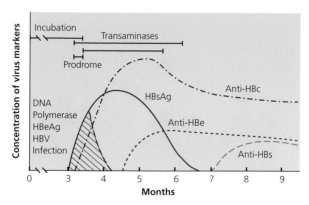

Figure 13.2 Typical course of an acute infection with hepatitis B virus (HBV). Ag, antigen; HBe, hepatitis B e; HBc, hepatitis B core; HBs, hepatitis B surface. (Courtesy of *British Journal of Hospital Medicine*.)

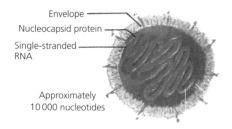

Figure 13.3 A hepatitis C virus (diameter 50–60 nm). (Courtesy of Ortho Diagnostic Systems.)

undergoing acute infection or to carriers with subliminal levels of hepatitis B surface antigen (HBsAg) in blood donations.

Screening for HBsAg is mandatory. Assays for antibody to hepatitis B core, HBc (total antibody and immunoglobulin M, IgM) are available for diagnosing acute hepatitis B infection. Assay for hepatitis B core (HBc) antibody should not replace that for HBsAg screening of donors; however in some countries both tests are done routinely on all blood units. In the UK only donors with a history of hepatitis or body piercing are tested for anti-HBc. Screening for the delta agent is unnecessary as delta depends on HBV to provide its surface antigen. Screening for antibody to HBsAg can be used to identify donors whose plasma is suitable for the preparation of hepatitis B immunoglobulin. In the UK, HBV is detected in approximately 1 in 25 000 donations overall, a lower rate than in the general population because individuals at high risk of having human immunodeficiency virus (HIV) and, concomitantly, HBV are now excluding themselves from donation. Vaccine is available for protecting HBV-negative recipients of the products of pooled plasma (e.g. immunodeficient patients on permanent IgG therapy) and for patients who need regular transfusions (e.g. those with thalassaemia). Vaccine escape mutants of HBV have been reported. This necessitates careful validation of HBsAg assays.

Hepatitis C virus

Hepatitis C virus (HCV) (Figure 13.3) is a flavivirus causing most (in some countries, all) non-A, non-B hepatitis. Antibody to this agent can be detected by an enzyme-linked immunosorbent assay (ELISA). This uses antigen cloned from plasma known to transmit non-A, non-B hepatitis together with synthetic HCV antigens in some systems.

There may be at least two different viruses that transmit non-A, non-B hepatitis. Assays have been developed in which cloned antigens or synthetic peptides can react with antibody to HCV. The virus is plasma borne and has some routes of transmission in common with HBV. The incubation period for hepatitis C is commonly from 6 to 12 weeks.

Some countries require the screening of blood donors for antibody to hepatitis B core (anti-HBc) and the measurement of alanine aminotransferase (ALT) activity as surrogate markers for non-A,

non-B hepatitis. Most donations exhibiting only one of these abnormal markers, however, do not transmit hepatitis C, so 'surrogate' screening leads to unnecessary wastage of blood donations. The main causes of increased ALT activity in British blood donors are obesity and alcohol consumption. Assays for hepatitis C antibody are used routinely to screen blood donations. Improved screening assays based on recombinant or synthetic antigens including viral core protein have been developed. Very occasionally HCV may be transmitted by blood from donors in the early stages of infection. Direct testing for HCV nucleic acid using the nucleic acid amplification technique (NAT) can detect infection during most of the 'window period' before seroconversion. In the UK, this is usually performed on pools of samples. HCV antigen detection is almost as sensitive as pooled NAT and is cheaper and more convenient. In England and Wales, where ELISA for anti-HCV as well as NAT for HCV genome are used, the current residual risk per donation of HCV infection is one in 30 million.

In the USA, before screening for HCV antibody was introduced, about 10% of transfusions caused significant increases in transaminase activity in recipients, and there were occasional cases of symptomatic hepatitis; this figure is now less than one in a million.

Acute infection is usually mild, but a proportion of patients do develop chronic liver disease. Confirmed rates of positivity for anti-HCV (and thus carrier rates) in UK new donors are approximately one in 2000. Modern methods of viral inactivation of plasma-derived factors VIII and IX will prevent transmission. Haemophiliacs who have received effectively inactivated factor VIII have proved negative for antibody to HCV, in contrast to those who received uninactivated concentrate, with a worldwide anti-HCV prevalence greater than 70%, a prevalence similar to that in intravenous drug users. In the UK, haemophiliacs are no longer treated with plasma-derived products; they all receive recombinant coagulation factors.

Another flavivirus distantly related to HCV has been cloned and named hepatitis G virus (Box 13.1). However, it is not hepatotropic and the alternative name 'GB virus C' or GBV-C is more appropriate. Viraemia is present in ≥2% of blood donors and it has been shown to be transmissible by transfusion. It is considered to be non-pathogenic and is not causatively or predictively associated with elevated ALT levels in infected individuals. TTV and SEN-V are other cloned viruses initially thought to cause post-transfusion hepatitis. These circoviruses are considered non-pathogenic.

Hepatitis A and hepatitis E viruses only cause post-transfusion hepatitis very rarely because a carrier state does not occur.

Box 13.1 **The alphabet of viruses causing viral hepatitis**

- Hepatitis A virus: 'infectious hepatitis'
- Hepatitis B virus: 'serum hepatitis' (and variants)
- Hepatitis C virus: principal agent of non-A, non-B hepatitis
- Hepatitis D virus: delta agent
- Hepatitis E virus: enteric or epidemic
- 'Hepatitis F' virus: the initial report of 'fulminant' hepatitis caused by transfusion has never been subsequently corroborated
- ('Hepatitis G' virus: a non-hepatotrophic and non-pathogenic virus more appropriately referred to as GBV-C)

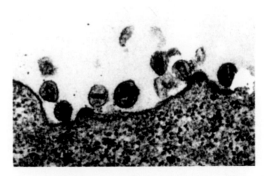

Figure 13.5 HIV-1 replicating in a lymphocytic leukaemia cell line culture. (Courtesy of Dr D. Robertson and Professor R.A. Weiss, Chester Beatty Laboratories, Institute of Cancer Research.)

Human immunodeficiency virus

HIV-1 (Figure 13.5) was transmitted by transfusion before screening for anti-HIV was introduced and before donors at high risk started excluding themselves from giving blood. HIV-2 occurs mainly in West Africa. Both are retroviruses, 100 nm in diameter, that carry their own RNA-dependent DNA polymerase (reverse transcriptase). Before screening was introduced, HIV had been transmitted by whole blood, red cell components, platelet concentrates and FFP. It can contaminate factor VIII and factor IX concentrates, but it can readily be inactivated chemically or by heat and modern concentrates do not transmit it. It has not been transmitted by albumin, immunoglobulins or antithrombin III. With current anti-HIV assays, the seroconversion period is rarely longer than 1 month, and a primary illness similar to glandular fever may occur during this time. The incubation period for the acquired immune deficiency syndrome (AIDS) is variable, with a likely median time of at least 7 years in adults (although the period is shorter for infants) (Figure 13.4).

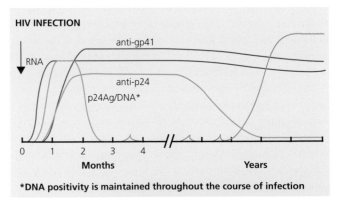

Figure 13.4 Sequence of events following human immunodeficiency virus (HIV) infection. (Courtesy of Abbott Diagnostics Ltd.)

Screening for HIV antibody is by an 'antiglobulin' or 'sandwich' ELISA, capture ELISA or, in some countries, gelatin particle or 'rapid' (e.g. dipstick) assays. 'Competitive' assays specifically for anti-HIV-1 have been superseded by assays that can detect both anti-HIV-1 and -2. In recent years 'combi' ELISAs that detect anti-HIV-1 and -2 together with HIV antigen in a single assay have reduced the window period of HIV infection to just a few days. Although some countries such as the USA and the UK employ NAT for HIV detection in addition to serological assays, the residual risk per donation for HIV in England and Wales, before NAT for HIV was introduced, was only one in 5 million because of the sensitivity of serological testing and the low incidence of HIV infection in donors. This low incidence of 'window period' infections is not the case in countries with high rates of HIV infection, such as Thailand and South Africa, where donation screening for South Africa, HIV antigen has detected several positive donors who had not yet developed anti-HIV.

Transmission of HIV by transfusion has been extremely rare since the introduction of screening. HIV antibody is found in one in 100 000 donations overall in the UK. The rate is significantly higher in new donors (one in 13 000) than in known donors (one in 176 000). 'Seroconverting' donations (those negative for HIV antibody but infectious because of recent infection) are therefore extremely rare. On only three occasions has a donation from a sero-negative donor been known to have transmitted HIV infection to 5 recipients in the UK since screening started in 1985. The virus can be inactivated in fractionated blood products by treatment with heat or chemicals, but components such as red cells or platelets cannot be heat treated. Methods for inactivating such cellular components are, however, being assessed, although so far they are logistically and financially demanding.

Adult T-cell leukaemia and human T-cell leukaemia virus

Human T-cell leukaemia virus type I (HTLV-I) is another pathogenic retrovirus (Figure 13.6). The clinical importance of HTLV-II is not clear; in the West it is associated with intravenous drug use and worldwide it has been found in a few cases of hairy cell leukaemia. Much of what has been reported as antibody to HTLV in the USA is likely to be antibody to HTLV-II. Both agents are associated with white cells and are not transmitted in plasma. The incubation period for adult T-cell leukaemia is about 20 years, but even then only about 1% of patients who are seropositive develop the disease. HTLV-I can also (rarely) cause tropical spastic paraparesis (also known as HTLV-I associated myelopathy or HAM), which has a much shorter

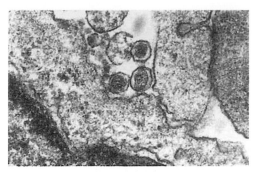

Figure 13.6 HTLV-I particles between cell membranes in a lymphocyte culture. (Courtesy of Dr D. Robertson and Professor R.A. Weiss, Chester Beatty Laboratories, Institute of Cancer Research.)

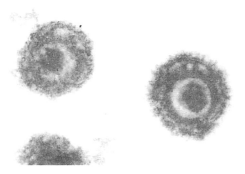

Figure 13.7 Cytomegalovirus particles showing characteristic herpes virus morphology (×100000). (Courtesy of J.E. Richmond, Public Health Laboratory Service Virus Reference Laboratory.)

incubation period than adult T-cell leukaemia. HTLV-I infection is endemic in the Caribbean, parts of Africa and Japan where 34% of the population are seropositive and where, before mandatory screening, transmission by transfusion was quite common.

In the UK the prevalence of anti-HTLV in blood donors varies from one in 20 000 to one in 80 000 or less, depending on the region. Blood donations are screened for HTLV antibodies using a very sensitive anti-HTLV assay on the pools of 48 samples prepared for HCV NAT testing.

Cytomegalovirus

Cytomegalovirus (CMV) (Figure 13.7) is a member of the herpes group of viruses, and latent infection of white cells in seropositive subjects may allow recrudescence of the virus. Viraemia in healthy donors is rare. The incubation period is up to 12 weeks, and blood transfusion can cause primary infection, reactivation of an endogenous latent infection, or reinfection with a different strain of the virus.

ELISAs are currently used for screening in the UK. Because severe (and sometimes fatal) CMV disease may occur only after transmission to immunosuppressed patients, selective screening of donors is sufficient to fulfil the demands of, in particular, CMV-negative recipients of bone marrow transplants and low birth weight premature infants. Granulocyte transfusions that are seropositive for CMV are especially likely to transmit the virus. About half of all donors in the UK are seropositive, and the rate increases

with age. Seropositivity also depends on the socioeconomic background of the subject and on the geographical location. However, only between 3% and 12% of donor units have the potential for transmitting the virus (especially, but not exclusively, if IgM CMV antibody is detectable), but there is no screening test to identify specifically those seropositive donors who are likely to be infectious. Components from which the white cells have been removed (i.e. leucodepleted units and frozen-thawed red cells) have been shown not to transmit CMV. Despite this, the current consensus in the UK is that, if anti-CMV screening is in place for blood for immunosuppressed recipients, it should continue, even if blood is leucodepleted. IgG given intravenously with antiviral agents helps to ameliorate the effects of CMV disease in immunosuppressed patients.

The recently described HHV 8 (human herpes virus 8), the causative agent of Kaposi's sarcoma, is white cell associated. It may therefore pose a potential risk for blood transfusion as transfusion has been implanted as a means of transmission.

Parvovirus B19

Although serum parvovirus is not usually pathogenic when transmitted by transfusion, it can lead to an aplastic crisis in a patient with chronic haemolytic anaemia (such as sickle cell anaemia) because of its inhibitory effect on red cell precursors. The risk of transmission by transfusion of non-pooled components is small because, as for hepatitis A, there is no carrier state and the period of viraemia is short in immunocompetent individuals. The titre of virus during the period of viraemia, however, is high and infectious units of plasma can contaminate batches of factor VIII; over 90% of recipients of untreated factor VIII are likely to be seropositive. Heat treatment of freeze-dried factor VIII at 80°C for 72 hours seems to inactivate most, if not all, of the virus. Some manufacturers of fractionated products therefore test pooled plasma with a low sensitivity B19 nucleic acid test, to exclude material containing high levels of viraemia.

Prion diseases

Despite continuing efforts to detect a nucleic acid involvement in prion disease (e.g. to help explain 'strain' differences), the infectious protein hypothesis remains the generally accepted model of pathogenesis. Prion transmission by transfusion has been clearly demonstrated in sheep and been strongly implicated in four human recipients. This important topic is covered in Chapter 14.

Conclusion

The number of viral infections that are potentially transmissible by blood transfusion seems daunting (see Table 13.1). Generally, persistent infections pose the major risk for transmission by transfusion. Acute infections only become a significant risk when their incidence is very high (e.g. West Nile virus in the USA). In the UK, however, the incidence of most of these infections in the general population is low. Most potential donors who are at high risk of transmitting infectious agents have voluntarily stopped giving blood, and donated blood is carefully screened, so the absolute numbers of infectious complications of blood transfusion are minute as demonstrated by the UK haemovigilance surveillance, SHOT (Serious Hazards of Transfusion, see Chapter 18). The possible risk from high incidence pandemics of acute infections such as SARS (severe acute respiratory syndrome) – so far averted – or 'bird flu' (the H5N1 strain of avian influenza) remain theoretical. However, transient viraemia has been demonstrated for both of these infections, so the situation is monitored closely. If outbreaks of either agent were to occur the risk of infection from transfusion should be considered in the context of the very high rates of community-acquired infections predicted. A similar situation pertains for Chikungunya fever and Dengue viruses.

Patients are at much greater risk if they do not have transfusions when they genuinely need them than they are from the possible infectious complications of transfusion, particularly as physicians are now more aware of the risks and far more discerning in their prescription of blood or its components.

Further reading

Barbara JAJ, Regan FAM, Contreras MC, eds. *Transfusion Microbiology*. Cambridge University Press, Cambridge, 2008.

Mollison PL, Engelfiet CP, Contreras M. Infectious agents transmitted by transfusion. In: *Blood Transfusion in Clinical Medicine*, 10th edn. Blackwell Science, Oxford, 1997, pp. 509–557.

Wendel S, Barbara JAJ. In: Lozano M, Contreras M, Blajchman M (eds) *Global Perspectives in Transfusion Medicine*. AABB Press, Bethesda, MD, 2006, pp. 55–101.

CHAPTER 14

Variant Creutzfeldt–Jakob Disease and its Impact on the UK Blood Supply

Patricia Hewitt, James Ironside and Marcela Contreras

OVERVIEW

- The prevalence of variant Creutzfeldt–Jakob disease (vCJD) infection in the population is unknown, but the number of cases of clinical disease has been falling since 1990.
- There is evidence that vCJD has been transmitted through blood transfusion from asymptomatic donors prior to development of clinical disease.
- Precautionary measures to reduce the risk of transmission through blood transfusion include donor selection measures (e.g. exclusion of transfused individuals as blood donors) and measures to reduce the prion load in blood (e.g. leucodepletion).
- Further measures designed to reduce even further the risk of vCJD transmission through blood transfusion (blood screening tests and prion-reduction filters) are under development.
- Measures to reduce the risk of transmission, other than blood processing methods, inevitably lead to a loss of donors or donations. Blood processing methods may lead to a reduction in red cell content of donations, also leading to a need for increased supply of blood donations.

Table 14.1 Classification of human prion diseases.

Sporadic disorders of unknown aetiology
- Sporadic Creutzfeldt–Jakob disease (CJD)
- Sporadic fatal insomnia

Familial disorders (associated with PRNP mutations or insertions)
- Familial CJD
- Gerstmann–Straussler–Scheinker disease
- Fatal familial insomnia

Acquired disorders

Transmission from human to human
- Kuru (transmitted by ritualistic endocannibalism)
- Iatrogenic CJD (transmitted by contaminated neurosurgical instruments and electrodes, corneal and dura mater grafts and pituitary hormone extracts)
- Iatrogenic variant CJD (transmitted by blood transfusion)

Transmission from bovine to human
- Variant CJD (most likely by the consumption of BSE-contaminated meat products)

BSE, bovine spongiform encephalopathy.

Prion diseases

Prion diseases (also known as transmissible spongiform encephalopathies or TSEs) are a group of fatal neurodegenerative diseases occurring in humans and other mammals (reviewed by Prusiner 2004). In humans, prion diseases occur in three major groups (Table 14.1), which represent sporadic, acquired or genetic forms of the diseases. Prion diseases are transmissible with prolonged incubation periods that in humans can reach several decades. Although the precise nature of the transmissible agents responsible for these diseases is uncertain, there is increasing evidence to support the prion hypothesis, which states that the transmissible agent or prion is devoid of nucleic acid and is composed mainly of an abnormal isoform of the prion protein (PrP^{Sc}). The normal form of the prion protein (PrP^{c}) is expressed in many tissues in the body of the general population and occurs at highest levels in neurons within the central nervous system (CNS).

A number of factors have been identified that influence the efficiency of transmission of prions, including:
- the route of transmission (intracerebral inoculation is most efficient)
- the amount of infected material inoculated
- host genetic susceptibility (see below).

Asymptomatic infection (or a "carrier state") has been recognized experimentally for many years and has been identified more recently in humans.

The commonest form of human prion disease is the sporadic form of Creutzfeldt–Jakob disease (sCJD), which occurs most commonly in the seventh decade of life. The clinical features are those of a rapidly progressive dementia with a range of other neurological abnormalities including visual abnormalities and movement disorders (particularly ataxia and myoclonus), resulting in death around 4 months after the disease onset. sCJD occurs as a worldwide disorder affecting around one patient per million of the population each year.

Although rare, prion diseases have caught the public attention in recent years due to the emergence of new forms of prion disease, bovine spongiform encephalopathy (BSE) and variant

ABC of Transfusion, 4th edition, 2009. Edited by Marcela Contreras. © 2009 Blackwell Publishing, ISBN: 978-1-4051-5646-2.

Creutzfeldt–Jakob disease (vCJD). BSE (or 'mad cow disease') occurred as an epidemic in UK cattle in the 1980s and 1990s, and during that time a very large number of BSE-infected cattle carcasses would have been likely to enter the human food chain, giving rise to possible human infection with BSE through contaminated meat products.

In order to address the question of transmission of BSE to humans, surveillance of all forms of Creutzfeldt–Jakob disease was reinstigated in the UK in 1990, with a National CJD Surveillance Unit established in Edinburgh. In 1996 the unit reported a series of 10 patients in the UK who were suffering from a novel form of prion disease, now known as vCJD (Will et al. 1996). In contrast to sCJD, the age of disease onset is much younger (mean 28 years), with a longer duration of illness (mean 14 months) and a characteristic clinical course beginning with psychiatric abnormalities (anxiety, depression, personality change), sensory abnormalities, ataxia, myoclonus and progressive dementia. Since then, experimental transmission studies to mice have shown that the prion responsible for vCJD has identical properties to the BSE prion, indicating that vCJD is the 'human form of BSE' (Bruce et al. 1997). A comparison of sCJD and vCJD is summarized in Table 14.2.

vCJD is also unique amongst other prion diseases in that PrP^{Sc} accumulation and infectivity can be readily detected outside the CNS, particularly in lymphoid tissues, where there is an accumulation of PrP^{Sc} within germinal centres that co-localizes to follicular dendritic cells. Experimental studies in animal models have indicated that the replication of the prion agents can occur at these sites, prior to neuroinvasion and well before the onset of neurological symptoms. The accumulation of PrP^{Sc} in lymphoid tissues prior to the onset of clinical disease in vCJD has also allowed the use of tonsil biopsy as an aid to premortem diagnosis in some patients.

Transmission of vCJD by blood

The widespread tissue distribution of PrP^{Sc} and infectivity in vCJD has given rise to concerns that infectivity might also be present in blood. Studies in sheep infected with BSE have demonstrated transmission of infection by blood transfusion from donor sheep during the incubation stage of the disease. In 1997, a joint study was set up between the UK blood services and the UK National CJD Surveillance Unit, to examine whether there is any link between blood transfusion and Creutzfeldt–Jakob disease (Hewitt et al. 2006). By early 2007, this study had identified four incidents of apparent transmission of vCJD infectivity by transfusion of non-leucodepleted red blood cells from three different donors who all subsequently died from vCJD. The first case occurred in a patient who developed the clinical features of vCJD 6.5 years after transfusion, and the second occurred in a patient who died around 5 years after transfusion but without clinical features of vCJD. However, PrP^{Sc} accumulation was detected biochemically and by immunohistochemistry in lymphoid tissues (but not in the CNS) in this recipient, indicating an asymptomatic or preclinical infection. The third and fourth cases occurred around 8 years following transfusion, resulting in a clinical illness with the diagnostic features of vCJD.

All patients with the clinical features of vCJD to date (including the first, third and fourth transfusion-associated cases) have been methionine homozygotes at codon 129 in the prion protein gene (*PRNP*) (Table 14.3). The incidence of vCJD has declined in the UK from a peak in 2000 (Figure 14.1), but it remains to be established whether BSE infection in other human PRNP genotypes will result in a similar clinical and neuropathological phenotype to vCJD, hence continuing surveillance is required.

Impact of vCJD on the UK blood supply

Although first described only 10 years ago, vCJD has already had a significant impact on the UK blood supply. The direct impact of vCJD in relation to the UK blood supply is in two main areas–blood donors and blood donations. A third area which has also felt the impact is blood usage.

Table 14.2 Comparison of sporadic Creutzfeldt–Jakob disease (sCJD) and variant Creutzfeldt–Jakob disease (vCJD).

	sCJD	vCJD
Distribution	Worldwide	UK, with smaller numbers in 10 other countries
Incidence	One per million population per annum	Since 1996, 165 cases in UK (incidence in decline since 1999)
Mean age at onset (years)	65	28
Mean duration of illness (months)	4	14
Aetiology	Unknown	Likely dietary exposure to BSE
PRNP codon 129 genotypes affected	MM, MV, VV	MM (all clinical cases so far)
Infectivity present outside CNS	Infrequent and at low levels	Present in lymphoid tissues and peripheral nervous system
Associated with transmission by blood transfusion	No	Yes (non-leucodepleted red blood cells)

BSE, bovine spongiform encephalopathy; CNS, central nervous system; M, methionine; V, valine.

Table 14.3 Prion protein gene (*PRNP*) polymorphisms and human prion diseases.

	PRNP codon 129 polymorphism frequency (%)		
	MM	*MV*	*VV*
Normal population	38	51	11
sCJD	71	15	14
vCJD	100	–	–

M, methionine; V, valine.

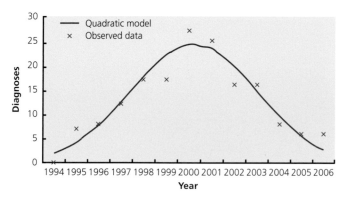

Figure 14.1 Quadratic exponential model for vCJD diagnoses incidence trend.

Market research and donor surveys have been used in an effort to predict some of the impacts of vCJD on the blood supply. These initiatives, together with modelling of likely future supply and demand, help to inform planning and communications with donors.

Impact of vCJD on blood donors

New donor selection criteria have been introduced with the aim of reducing the risk of collecting blood from a donor incubating vCJD. These new criteria have reduced the number of available blood donors and donations. The most important of the new criteria is the exclusion of individuals who have received a blood transfusion within the UK since 1980. Preliminary work, prior to implementation in April 2004, suggested that the impact would be to reduce the number of available blood donations by between 3% and 6%, depending on how the rule was applied (only to those with a certain history of transfusion, or also to those with a possible history). Without compensatory recruitment efforts, such a loss would have created severe difficulties in maintaining a blood supply.

There is a risk that some decisions in relation to blood safety/risk reduction could lead to disaffected donors, who stop donating even though not affected. An example is the donor notification exercise carried out over the summer of 2005, when just over 100 donors were notified that they were now considered at risk of vCJD 'for public health purposes' because their donations were transfused to a recipient who later developed vCJD. A small number of unaffected donors expressed concerns over this decision and indicated that they would consider whether to continue as a donor in future.

There is no current evidence of a significant problem, but other decisions might, if unpopular with donors, lead to a loss in willing donors.

Future initiatives, such as a possible blood screening test for vCJD, will inevitably lead to a loss of blood donors. Any screening test will produce a number of reactive results. A blood donation producing repeatedly reactive results cannot be used. There will therefore be less available donations. Confirmation of screening results is likely to present challenges, especially in the early days of use of a screening test. It may be the case that there is no practical confirmatory test available, in which case donors whose blood produces repeat reactive tests may be unable to continue donating at all since it is unacceptable to keep taking donations that cannot be used. Furthermore, donors may not want to be tested, and may stop donating when, and if, a test is introduced. Although there is little evidence to suggest that this will happen, it remains an unknown.

Impact of vCJD on blood donations

Universal leucodepletion of all blood components was introduced in the UK in the late 1990s and fully implemented by 1999 as a measure for reducing risk of vCJD transmission. This intervention inevitably added to the cost of blood components. It is too early to know whether it has been effective for the risk of vCJD transmission, but there may be other, non-vCJD, benefits such as reduction in alloimmunization to human leucocyte antigens and fewer febrile non-haemolytic transfusion reactions.

There is currently no blood screening test available for evidence of vCJD infection, but several commercial companies are working to develop a test that could be applied to blood donations. A test will inevitably lead to a loss of donations through repeat reactive results (whether or not confirmed). It is far too early to know the rates of repeat reactivity, false positivity and true positivity which might be expected. At present there is no immediate prospect of confirmatory tests or alternative assays that could allow reinstatement of donors with falsely reactive screening tests, such as happens currently for hepatitis B, C and human immunodeficiency virus (HIV).

Prion removal filters are being developed for red cells as an approach to reducing the risk of transmission of prions by blood transfusion. Filters would be expected to lead to an increase in red cell losses, possibly increasing the number of units of red cells needed for a therapeutic dose. This in turn would require increased collection targets, and result in increased donor exposure for recipients.

Where alternative supplies exist, blood components may be imported from areas of the world with little or no evidence of vCJD. This is already the case in the UK for fresh frozen plasma for fractionation and for transfusion to children. Knock-on effects include added cost, wastage of large volumes of UK plasma exposure to other (different) risks presented by a non-UK donor base, and more complicated inventory and prescription procedures.

Impact of vCJD on blood usage

When HIV first became a transfusion issue, blood usage decreased in some areas through increased recipient awareness, and demands for alternative strategies. In the UK, there has been a big push for 'better use of blood' over the last 4–5 years which is now beginning to bear fruit (see Chapter 18). It is not totally clear whether the reduction in use is a vCJD effect, or is primarily due to cost pressures or other issues (e.g. changes in surgical and anaesthetic techniques).

Every new intervention has a cost. The introduction of a further test for blood donations will inevitably increase the cost of blood – through a direct effect (cost of the test kit and any additional staff) and an indirect effect (cost of wasted donations, cost of additional recruitment efforts to replace lost donations/donors).

Further reading

Bruce E, Will RG, Ironside JW, et al. Transmissions to mice indicate that 'new variant' CJD is caused by the BSE agent. *Nature* 1997; **389**: 498–501.

Hewitt PE, Llewelyn CA, Mackenzie J, Will RG. Creutzfeldt–Jakob disease and blood transfusion: results of the UK Transfusion Medicine Epidemiological Review study. *Vox Sanguinis* 2006; **91**: 221–30.

Prusiner SB. An introduction to prion biology and diseases. In: Crotty D & Schaefer S, eds. *Prion Biology and Diseases*, 2nd edn. Cold Spring Harbor Laboratory Press, New York, 2004: 1–87.

Will RG, Ironside JW, Zeidler M, et al. A new variant Creutzfeldt–Jakob disease in the UK. *Lancet* 1996; **347**: 921–5.

CHAPTER 15

Risks of Transfusion in the Context of Haemovigilance: SHOT – the UK Haemovigilance System

Dorothy Stainsby, Hannah Cohen and Brian McClelland

OVERVIEW

- Haemovigilance is the systematic surveillance of adverse reactions and events relating to blood transfusion.
- Haemovigilance data are used to drive improvements in safety throughout the transfusion chain.
- The Serious Hazards of Transfusion (SHOT) scheme is the UK's haemovigilance system.
- SHOT data since 1996 show that 'incorrect blood component transfused' (IBCT) is consistently the most frequently reported hazard, and can have fatal consequences.
- The most common error resulting in IBCT is failure to carry out final identification checks next to the patient immediately before the blood is given.

Haemovigilance is generally defined as the systematic surveillance of adverse reactions and events relating to blood transfusion. Its aim is to accumulate evidence on the relative risks of blood transfusion that can be used to:

- drive improvements in hospital transfusion practice
- support development of national guidelines and local protocols
- inform blood safety policy decisions at the national level
- educate clinicians who use blood, and patients who receive it.

The Serious Hazards of Transfusion (SHOT) scheme was established in 1996. It is UK-wide, professionally led and affiliated to the Royal College of Pathologists. Participation in the SHOT scheme is a requirement of the Chief Medical Officers' Better Blood Transfusion initiatives and is a standard for compliance with the Clinical Negligence Scheme for Trusts (CNST) in England. The scheme is confidential and complies with UK legislation on data protection. The most recent SHOT data can be found on their website, www.shotuk.org.

How SHOT works

When an adverse transfusion reaction or an error in the transfusion process occurs, it should be reported without delay to a member of the hospital transfusion team (HTT). This team will usually include a consultant haematologist with responsibility for transfusion, a transfusion practitioner, and the blood transfusion laboratory manager (or senior biomedical scientist). The HTT is a source of expertise and advice on investigation and management of transfusion problems, and will ensure that untoward incidents are reported appropriately. Those reportable to SHOT are summarized in Table 15.1.

Reporting to SHOT is electronic, via the Serious Blood Reactions and Events (SABRE) on-line haemovigilance reporting system developed by the Medicines and Healthcare Products Regulatory Agency (MHRA) to meet the requirements of the Blood Safety and Quality Regulations 2005 (see Chapter 20). Reporters are asked to complete a comprehensive questionnaire; this is then scrutinized by a member of the SHOT Working Group. This group is responsible for extracting the data and using it to compile the annual report and to formulate recommendations (Figure 15.1).

What have we learned from SHOT?

The total number of incidents reported to SHOT between 1996 and 2005 is shown in Figure 15.2. It is very likely that this is an underestimate, as, although 99% of NHS Trusts claim to participate in SHOT, only 69% of eligible hospitals reported incidents and/or near misses in 2005 and the rate of reporting varies widely. Case reporting depends on clinical vigilance and awareness, an open culture in which reporting is encouraged, and the resources to investigate and report cases.

During the same time period, 30 million blood components were issued by the UK blood services. Data from the National Blood Service (NBS)/NHS Blood Stocks Management Scheme indicates that the number of red cells transfused is about 5% less than those issued. There are no published data on numbers of patients transfused or the number of transfusion episodes, and risk estimates can only be based on the number of units transfused, rather than the number of patients exposed to the risk. Whilst acknowledging these limitations of both numerator and denominator data, it is possible to estimate the observed frequency of serious transfusion hazards, as shown in Table 15.2.

Such estimates can be useful when discussing the relative risk and benefits of transfusion for an individual patient, or when

---

ABC of Transfusion, 4th edition, 2009. Edited by Marcela Contreras. © 2009 Blackwell Publishing, ISBN: 978-1-4051-5646-2.

Table 15.1 Categories of adverse reactions and events reportable to Serious Hazards of Transfusion (SHOT).

Category	SHOT definition
Incorrect blood component ('wrong blood') transfused (IBCT)	Patient transfused with a blood component or product which did not meet the appropriate requirement or was intended for another patient
Acute transfusion reaction	Adverse reactions occurring up to 24 hours following transfusion, excluding those due to IBCT
Delayed transfusion reaction	Clinical adverse reactions (not simple serological reactions) occurring more than 24 hours following transfusion of blood components
Transfusion-related acute lung injury	Acute dyspnoea with hypoxia and pulmonary infiltrates within 6 hours of transfusion, with no other apparent cause
Transfusion-associated graft-versus-host disease	Development of the classical symptoms of fever, rash, liver dysfunction and pancytopenia occurring 1–6 weeks post-transfusion, without other apparent cause. Diagnosis supported by skin/marrow biopsy appearances and/or presence of circulating donor lymphocytes
Post-transfusion purpura	Thrombocytopenia 5–12 days post-transfusion associated with antibodies in the patient directed against the HPA (human platelet antigen) system
Transfusion-transmitted infection	Post-transfusion infection in which: • the recipient had no evidence of infection pre-transfusion and either • at least one component was donated by a donor with evidence of the same transmissible infection or • at least one component was shown to have been contaminated with the infective agent
Near miss event	Any error which, if undetected, could result in the determination of a wrong blood group, or issue, collection or administration of an incorrect, inappropriate or unsuitable component but which was recognized before transfusion took place
Adverse event or reaction associated with autologous transfusion	Includes preoperative donation and blood salvage

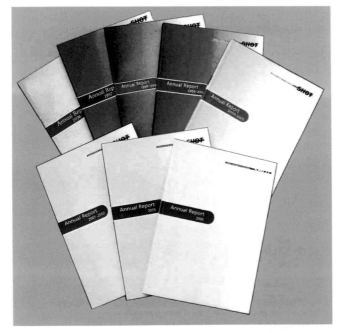

Figure 15.1 The covers of eight SHOT reports from 1996 to 2004.

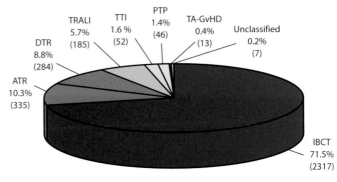

Figure 15.2 Total incidents reported to SHOT, 1996–2005 ($n = 3239$). ATR, acute transfusion reaction; DTR, delayed transfusion reaction; IBCT, incorrect blood component transfused; PTP, post-transfusion purpura; TA-GvHD, transfusion-associated graft-versus-host disease; TRALI, transfusion-related acute lung injury; TTI, transfusion-transmitted infection.

Making transfusion safer

Transfusion-associated mortality and morbidity between 1996 and 2005 is shown in Table 15.3. SHOT defines major morbidity as one or more of the following:
• a requirement for intensive care admission and/or ventilation
• acute renal failure
• major haemorrhage due to transfusion-related coagulopathy
• intravascular haemolysis
• potential D sensitization of a female of childbearing potential

decisions are to be made about allocation of resources for blood safety. It is salutary to compare them with the very small residual risks of transfusion-transmitted viral infections for which blood is routinely tested (see Chapter 13).

Table 15.2 Frequency of reported serious hazards of blood transfusion in the UK estimated using data to 2004 (not all incident types are included).

Event	Number of incidents reported	Frequency of reported events per 100 000 components issued
Incorrect blood component transfused (IBCT)	1832	7
ABO incompatible transfusions (all components – included in IBCT)	249	1
Death as a result of IBCT	20	0.07
Transfusion-related acute lung injury (TRALI)	162	0.6
Fatal TRALI	36	0.1
Acute transfusion reaction (ATR)	267	1
Transfusion-transmitted infection (including bacterial)	49	0.2
Total adverse reactions/events	2630	10
Total transfusion-related deaths	100	0.4

Table 15.3 Transfusion-associated mortality and morbidity, 1996–2005.

	Total	IBCT	ATR	DTR	PTP	TA-GvHD	TRALI	TTI
Death definitely attributed to transfusion (imputability 3)	46	7	2	6	1	13	8	9
Death probably attributed to transfusion (imputability 2)	13	3	4	1	0	0	5	0
Death possibly attributed to transfusion (imputability 1)	46	12	7	1	1	0	25	0
Subtotal 1	105	22	13	8	2	13	38	9
Major morbidity* probably or definitely attributed to transfusion reaction (imputability 2/3)	295	93	13	29	13	0	110	37
Minor or no morbidity as a result of transfusion reaction	2240	2191	306	246	31	0	37	6
Subtotal 2	3112	2284	319	275	44	0	147	43
Outcome unknown	15	11	3	1	0	0	0	0
Total†	3232	2317	335	284	46	13	185	52

ATR, acute transfusion reaction; DTR, delayed transfusion reaction; IBCT, incorrect blood component transfused; TA-GvHD, transfusion-associated graft-versus-host disease; TRALI, transfusion-related acute lung injury; TTI, transfusion-transmitted infection.
* Excludes seven unclassifiable cases.
† Excludes three cases reported prior to inception of SHOT.

• persistent viral infection
• acute symptomatic infection (viral, bacterial or protozoal).
Other sections of this book highlight the immunological and infectious risks of transfusion and describe the measures taken in the UK to reduce these risks. Continuing SHOT data will be essential to monitor the impact of initiatives such as those aimed at reducing bacterial contamination of platelets (see Chapter 12) and the implementation of male-only FFP to reduce the risk of transfusion-related acute lung injury (TRALI), currently the leading cause of transfusion-related mortality and morbidity (see Chapter 11).

The next section will therefore focus on incorrect blood component transfused – the most frequently reported transfusion hazard, comprising 71.5% of reported events and accounting in whole or in part for reports of 22 deaths and 94 cases of major morbidity in the UK over a period of 9 years.

Incorrect blood component transfused: what goes wrong and how it can be prevented

The most serious consequence of an error in blood administration is a fatal ABO incompatible transfusion (Figure 15.3). This may be the end result of adverse events such as patient misidentification, sample mislabelling, laboratory errors, collection of the wrong component from the blood bank, and/or administration to the wrong patient. Analysis of these events (Figure 15.4) reveals that in

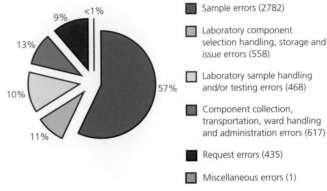

Figure 15.5 Distribution of errors in near miss reports, 1997–2005 (*n* = 4861).

SATURDAY, OCTOBER 10, 1998

Daily Mail

NAMES MIX-UP KILLS PATIENT

Tragedy of blood blunder

By MICHAEL SEAMARK

A HOSPITAL patient died after a tragically simple mix-up over names.

Ward staff twice gave Philip James blood labelled for a patient called James Philip.

The blood was a different group to 75-year old Mr James's, his body rejected it and he suffered a fatal heart attack.

Without the transfusions, an inquest heard yesterday, the pensioner would almost certainly have recovered satisfactorily from his operation.

Figure 15.3 The most serious consequence of a 'wrong blood' error.

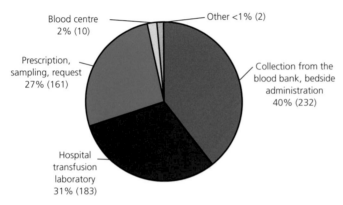

Figure 15.4 Where errors occur in the transfusion chain: distribution of 588 errors identified in 348 IBCT (incorrect blood component transfused) reports analysed in 2003.

approximately half of cases there is more than one error, that 70% of errors take place in clinical areas and 30% in hospital transfusion laboratories, and that failure of the final patient identification check contributes to 30% of cases.

A blood sample for pre-transfusion testing that has been taken from the wrong patient is usually detectable by the laboratory if the patient has been previously tested and the results are accessed. These errors result in relatively few reports to SHOT. But clinical audit reveals that in one in 2000 samples sent to laboratories the blood in the tube does not match the patient details, and reports to SHOT of near misses reveal the true extent of sample misidentification (Figure 15.5).

Contributory factors to errors include: labelling the sample away from the bedside, failure to positively check patient identity, use of preprinted 'addressograph' labels (proscribed by the British Committee for Standards in Haematology, BCSH), phlebotomist distracted or multitasking, and sharing of tasks (e.g. handing over an unlabelled sample to be labelled by another person).

Poor techniques in blood sampling for diagnostic investigations may give rise to inappropriate transfusions, sometimes with disastrous consequences. Successive SHOT reports include cases where

blood has been taken from a vein into which an infusion is running, or has been allowed to settle in a syringe, resulting in an erroneous haemoglobin result and an inappropriate decision to transfuse, sometimes with fatal results. All staff undertaking phlebotomy must receive training and competence assessment. Hospital policies should state that blood samples must be taken from a free flowing venepuncture site, the tube filled to capacity and adequately mixed. The phlebotomist must complete the tube label before leaving the patient, checking verbally with the patient that the identification details are correct and against the ID wristband or equivalent.

The most critical stage in the transfusion chain, accounting for 40% of errors, is the collection of the blood from the blood bank or satellite refrigerator and its administration to the patient.

Consistently the commonest error in reports of 'wrong blood' to SHOT is a failure to carry out a final patient identification check. 'Checking' blood away from the bedside against paperwork such as a compatibility label, prescription chart or patient notes, whilst omitting to check against the patient wristband is a recipe for catastrophe! It cannot be emphasized too strongly that all transfused patients *must* be identified by a correct wristband, or an alternative form of identification that conforms to national standards, and this *must* be used to identify the patient before administering blood components (Figure 15.6). Adherence to standards for patient identification will also reduce errors in other areas of health care such as drug administration.

Transfusion errors can cause harm to patients in other ways than ABO incompatibility. Certain groups of patients (notably neonates and children, immunosuppressed patients and patients with red cell alloantibodies) have special and sometimes complex transfusion requirements. Failure to comply with transfusion guidelines (e.g. BCSH guidelines on indications for irradiation of components, and those on the provision of blood for neonates and children) can result in the transfusion of unsuitable blood components and expose patients to risk of harm. National guidelines should be translated into accessible local protocols supported by training and education, and expert advice from a haematologist should always be available.

Clinicians prescribing blood should ensure that all relevant information about the patient's transfusion history, reason for transfusion and diagnosis are communicated to the laboratory

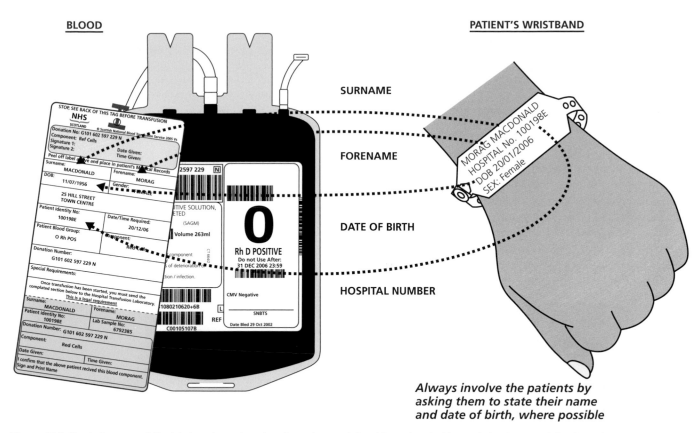

BLOOD

PATIENT'S WRISTBAND

SURNAME

FORENAME

DATE OF BIRTH

HOSPITAL NUMBER

Always involve the patients by asking them to state their name and date of birth, where possible

Figure 15.6 Check the compatibility label on the pack against the patient's wristband (reproduced with permission from McClelland 2007).

on the appropriate form. This is of particular importance when patient care is shared and the patient's laboratory record may not be available.

The role of information technology

Information technology can support the transfusion process at all stages in the chain. Systems are available to print sample labels at the bedside, to control the release of blood components from the blood bank and to ensure correct bedside administration. Laboratory information technology systems are capable of 'flagging' the patient's transfusion history and special requirements, and supporting the selection and issue of the correct blood components.

A developing safety culture

Successive SHOT reports have encouraged open reporting of adverse events and 'near misses' in a supportive, learning culture, vigilance in hospital transfusion practice and evaluation of information technology to support the transfusion process. The importance of education and training has been emphasized. SHOT has no power to implement change, but exerts its influence through the professional bodies represented on the steering group and by feedback, education and lobbying. The national, regional and hospital transfusion committees, supported by the UK blood services, provide a network for the development and dissemination

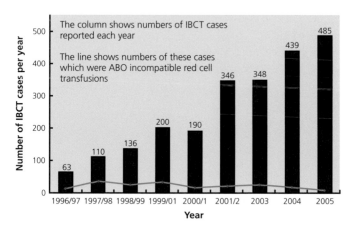

Figure 15.7 ABO incompatible transfusions, 1996–2005, in the context of increasing numbers of IBCT (incorrect blood component transfused) reports. A developing safety culture?

of good practice. Collaboration between SHOT, the Chief Medical Officer for England's National Blood Transfusion Committee and the National Patient Safety Agency, has resulted in an initiative aimed at reducing ABO incompatible transfusions by improving bedside practice. A further initiative is required to improve laboratory practice.

Figure 15.7 shows that, against a background of ever-increasing vigilance and improved reporting of adverse events, the number of ABO incompatible transfusions is decreasing; an indication of an emerging safety culture that bodes well for patient safety. This must be nurtured by ensuring that hospitals can guarantee professional accountability, implement education programmes and assess and document competency.

The need for an overarching view of transfusion risks

From the inception of SHOT, a key recommendation has been a call for an overarching body with the expertise and remit to assess and prioritize transfusion risks. Transfusion safety is emotive, controversial and politically sensitive, and there is a need for objectivity and scientific rigour when allocating resources to safety initiatives.

Users of blood can contribute to transfusion safety by ensuring that robust protocols are in place, that all staff prescribing, handling and administering blood are competent to do so, and, above all, that blood freely and generously donated is used appropriately according to clinical need.

Further reading

British Committee for Standards in Haematology guidelines, www.bcsh-guidelines.com.

Kleinman S, Chan P, Robillard P. Risks associated with transfusion of cellular blood components in Canada. *Transfusion Medicine Reviews* 2003; **17**(2): 120–62.

McClelland DBL, ed. *Handbook of Transfusion Medicine*, 4th edn. UK Blood Services, London, 2007.

SHOT reports, www.shotuk.org.

Stainsby D, Jones H, Asher D et al. Serious hazards of transfusion. A decade of Haemovigilance in the UK. *Transfusion Medicine Reviews* 2006; **20**(4): 273–82.

Stainsby D, Russell J, Cohen H, Lilleyman J. Reducing adverse events in blood transfusion. *British Journal of Haematology* 2005; **131**: 1–8.

Taylor C, Jones H, Davies T et al. (2008) SHOT Annual Report 2007. ISBN 978-09558648-0-3.

CHAPTER 16

Alternatives to Allogeneic Blood Transfusion

Dafydd Thomas and Beverley Hunt

OVERVIEW

- Autologous transfusion can complement a blood conservation programme.
- Better preoperative assessment helps minimize allogeneic transfusion.
- Red cell salvage is now the most commonly used form of autologous transfusion in the UK.
- Local audit of surgical activity and the need for allogeneic blood transfusion can help modulate blood conservation planning.
- An integrated care pathway can help coordinate the multidisciplinary perioperative approach.

There are a number of options available as transfusion alternatives. The successful avoidance of allogeneic transfusion will depend on whether the anaemia requiring treatment is chronic or acute and whether it is due to an underlying disease, to chemotherapeutic intervention or to trauma or surgery (Table 16.1). Current clinical practice in the UK is struggling to provide optimal preoperative preparation for patients. A suggested algorithm is highlighted in Figure 16.1.

The one area where the use of allogeneic blood transfusion has decreased significantly in recent years, in the UK, is in the treatment of acute perioperative anaemia. This has been achieved by a number of different strategies, all of which contribute to the overall aim of blood conservation, both of the patient's own blood and of allogeneic blood supplies. Measures that can be employed to minimize or eliminate the need for allogeneic transfusion during the perioperative period are addressed here. The most significant change in practice has been the acceptance by clinicians that withholding of allogeneic blood transfusion during this period, until there are signs or symptoms of anaemia, appears to be safe and results in a significant decrease in allogeneic transfusion. Controlled anaemia during the perioperative period does not increase mortality and patients soon recover, replenishing their own blood in the weeks following surgery. Published guidelines vary, but almost all state that transfusion to patients with a haemoglobin over 70 g/L is

ABC of Transfusion, 4th edition, 2009. Edited by Marcela Contreras. © 2009 Blackwell Publishing, ISBN: 978-1-4051-5646-2.

Table 16.1 Causes of anaemia that might require transfusion.

Acute	Chronic
Trauma	Dietary iron deficiency
Surgical loss	Malignancy
Chemotherapy	Infectious diseases
Gastrointestinal bleeding	Parasitic diseases (e.g. malaria)
Pregnancy	Thalassaemia, sickle cell disease

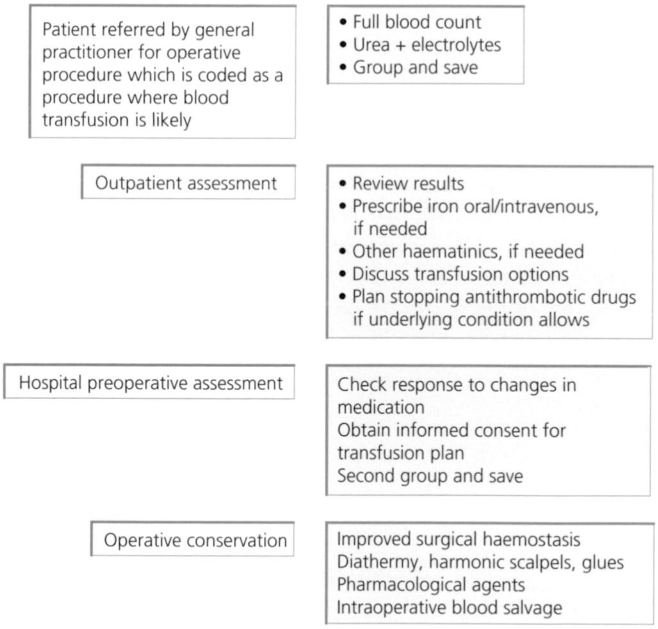

Figure 16.1 Preoperative algorithm to help aid perioperative blood conservation.

unnecessary if asymptomatic, with a slightly higher haemoglobin threshold for the elderly or those with cardiorespiratory disease.

The more widespread use of perioperative red cell salvage has helped reduce peri-surgical use of allogeneic red cells.

Preoperative preparation

A significant number of patients presenting for surgery are suffering from iron-deficiency anaemia. This may be as a result of their underlying illness or, as in a large number of elderly patients, as a result of poor diet. If noticed early in the preoperative period, oral iron is a very economic way of correcting this deficiency. Alternatively if time is short or there is an intolerance or non-compliance with oral iron, the use of intravenous iron sucrose appears very safe, efficacious and economic. If preoperative haemoglobin is increased, then there is a greater tolerance to blood loss.

Rational changes to preoperative medication

The cessation of anticoagulants prior to surgery is a long accepted alteration to a patient's usual medication. Stopping vitamin K antagonists and transfer to a low molecular weight heparin (LMWH) preoperatively is common practice. The heparin can then be stopped prior to surgery, so leaving only a narrow window when haemostasis is normal to allow surgical intervention, and restarting LMWH postoperatively. Regional anaesthesia can be undertaken providing thromboprophylactic LMWH is stopped 12 hours before. Other agents that may increase bleeding during the operative period can be safely stopped in some instances, providing it is not considered to increase the patient's risk of thromboembolism (e.g. clopidogrel, aspirin and other antiplatelet drugs). Aspirin needs to be stopped 7–10 days prior to surgery. Some patients with metal or drug eluting stents need to continue their dual antiplatelet therapy due to their high risk of rethrombosis; they thus have a high bleeding risk.

Operative haemostasis

Various surgical methods can be used to minimize operative blood loss. Operative haemostasis is the foundation upon which all other blood conservation methods are based. All other strategies are of little use if this has not been achieved.

The use of novel surgical techniques and instruments such as harmonic scalpels, water jet dissection, laparoscopic surgery and off-pump cardiac surgery all decrease the trauma to tissues and so may result in lower operative blood loss.

Autologous blood transfusion

In an attempt to further reduce the need for allogeneic blood, it is important that all measures to conserve the patient's own blood are taken. The use of perioperative blood salvage is currently the favoured method of autologous transfusion in the UK. Other methods include preoperative predeposit autologous donation (PAD), where a patient donates autologous blood in the weeks preceding surgery, and acute normovolaemic haemodilution, where venesection and collection of one in two units of blood is undertaken by the anaesthetist immediately prior to surgery. During acute normovolaemic haemodilution the blood loss is replaced with crystalloid or colloid solution to maintain isovolaemia and then the autologous blood is returned at the end of surgery.

These last two methods have recently been discouraged in the UK, due to the cost and wastage in PAD and lack of evidence of significant reduction in allogeneic red cell use in the latter. In addition, stored PAD presents a similar risk of an incorrect blood component being transfused as with allogeneic blood transfusion. The

demands on blood supplies may change in the future and both of these methods may be revisited. They both remain of value in specific situations, such as for patients with extremely rare blood groups requiring transfusions. For such patients, it is justifiable to keep their blood frozen in a cryoprotectant.

Red cell salvage techniques

These techniques may be performed during the surgical procedure or following surgery. The surgical wound drains (which collect blood that is usually discarded) may be used as a reservoir from which the patient's blood can be recycled. The collection to transfusion ratio is high, as only blood that is being lost is replaced. This latter fact helps to improve the cost effectiveness of perioperative techniques. The availability of cell salvage methods allows surgical blood ordering schedules (see Chapter 3) to be reduced, therefore decreasing blood bank work. There are two main techniques involved in perioperative salvage: (i) collection and reinfusion of wound drainage; and (ii) automated cell salvage.

Collection and reinfusion of wound drainage

The simplest method involves the collection of wound drainage blood and simple reinfusion. All these techniques consist of a main collection chamber that is connected to the wound drain via one port and a separate port to which an intravenous administration set can be attached (Figure 16.2). Reinfused blood passes through a

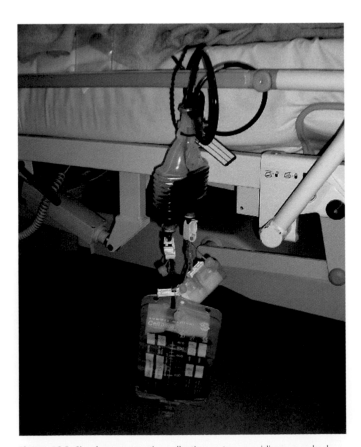

Figure 16.2 Simple postoperative collection system providing unwashed blood.

40 μm filter. No anticoagulant is added as the blood is assumed to be defibrinated, with clot formation having already occurred in the wound. The technique is probably best reserved for collection and reinfusion of blood in total knee replacement surgery and other joint replacement surgery.

Advantages

The main advantages of the simple collection systems are their relative ease of use and the avoidance of expensive and more complicated machines. The system can be used on the postoperative ward, where the collection and reinfusion of blood is under the care of the ward nursing staff.

Disadvantages

There are potentially more complications with these devices as unwashed blood is being reinfused. The subsequent administration of anticoagulant, cellular debris, free haemoglobin and activated leucocytes may lead to physiological problems if large amounts of this blood are transfused. Surprisingly, few adverse reports have been published. In practice the reinfusion of small volumes seems clinically acceptable.

The procedure is not recommended in cases where there is contamination of the salvaged product with bowel contents, malignant cells or amniotic fluid.

Automated cell salvage

The second method is regarded as the gold standard in operative recycling, where the collected blood is first filtered and then undergoes centrifugal separation, washing and resuspension in sterile saline. This produces a red cell product free of the contaminants mentioned above with a packed cell volume of 0.5. The recycling process may only take 8 minutes if the patient is bleeding large volumes.

Blood is collected from the surgical wound via a suction catheter (Figure 16.3). This catheter has two lumens, one to deliver heparinized saline (or other anticoagulant) (Figure 16.4) to the site of

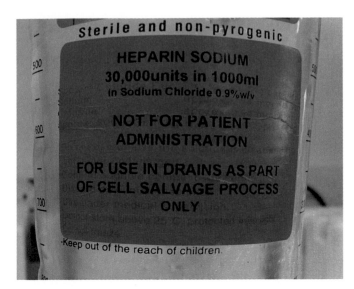

Figure 16.4 An example of pre-prepared heparinized saline wash solution.

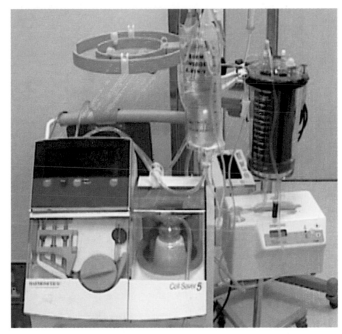

Figure 16.5 Cell salvage machine prepared for use.

haemorrhage, and the other to aspirate the already anticoagulated blood. The yield of red cells is improved if turbulence and red cell trauma is minimized. Red cell salvage is most successful when blood is aspirated from pooled blood rather than by constant suction from wound surfaces. The collected blood is then aspirated via a roller pump into the centrifuge bowl, further to passing through a 40 μm filter (Figure 16.5). After centrifugation, the supernatant is discarded and the red cells are washed and then suspended in normal saline for reinfusion (Figure 16.6).

Advantages

This technique provides washed red cells at a packed cell volume of 0.5. Disposable costs are minimized when blood salvage volumes

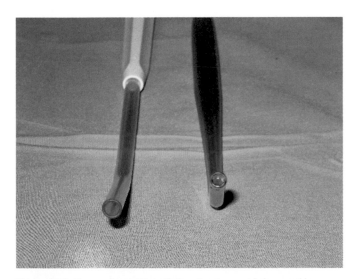

Figure 16.3 Atraumatic suction catheter showing a wide bore and less angulation to minimize turbulent flow of salvaged blood.

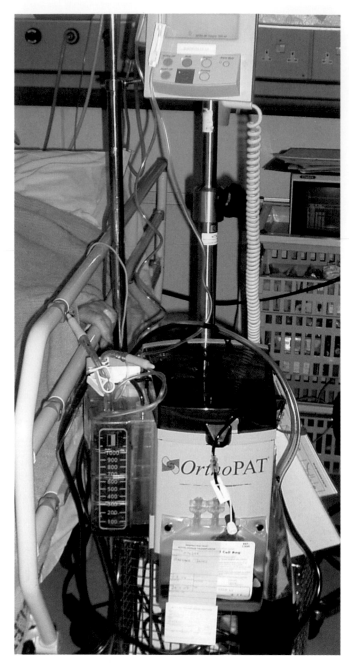

Figure 16.6 Compact machine for providing washed postoperative red cell salvage.

are large but probably become relatively cost effective for volumes of between 250 and 500 ml (equivalent to approximately 1 unit of packed cells). Fresh red cells are salvaged that have active oxygen carrying capacity. The alkaline pH of saved red cells minimizes acidosis associated with massive transfusion. There is no risk of hyperkalaemia as red cell ionic pumps remain active and K^+ remains within the red cells. The free haemoglobin levels are very low when compared with stored allogeneic red cells or simple reinfusion techniques. There remains a necessity to fully label all saved blood to avoid incorrect blood being transfused, in spite of the close proximity of all salvaged blood to the patient and the lack of need for storage (Figures 16.6 and 16.7).

Disadvantages

The technique requires trained operators and automated equipment is expensive to purchase. The technique is not recommended in cases where there is contamination of the salvaged product with bowel contents, malignant cells or amniotic fluid.

However, the National Institute for Clinical Excellence has given guarded support to the use of red cell salvage in obstetrics when there is significant haemorrhage. In the case of surgical fields which may contain malignant cells, the use of cell salvage is left to the discretion of the surgeon.

Antifibrinolytics

Activation of fibrinolysis occurs during all forms of surgery. Antifibrinolytic drugs, such as tranexamic acid and aprotinin, block the breakdown of fibrin (Figure 16.8).

Tranexamic acid is a competitive inhibitor of plasmin and plasminogen, preventing plasmin binding to fibrin. The Horrow regime (10 mg/kg followed by 1 mg/kg/h) has been shown to reduce blood loss in cardiac surgery. Other studies have used boluses of up to 5 g per patient, in bleeding patients, with no ill effect. ε-aminocaproic acid is also a synthetic lysine analogue that has a potency 10-fold weaker than tranexamic acid.

Aprotinin is a broad-spectrum serine protease inhibitor isolated from bovine lung, and is a powerful antiplasmin agent. The 'high dose' regimen (2 M KIU to the patient and a cardiopulmonary bypass prime and an infusion of 500 000 KIU/h; K stands for Kallikrein) has been shown to reduce perioperative bleeding in open cardiac surgery. Lower doses do produce adequate antiplasmin effects, however. A dose of 2 M units is approved for the treatment of established hyperfibrinolysis.

The efficacy of antifibrinolytic agents in preventing blood loss in elective surgery, and especially in cardiac surgery, has been shown in numerous clinical trials. A Cochrane review suggested that, despite the theoretically greater potency of aprotinin, there was little clinical difference in efficacy between it and tranexamic acid. Given prophylactically perioperative in elective surgery, these drugs reduce the need for red cell transfusion by about 30%, saving about 1 unit of red cells in patients requiring transfusion. The efficacy of tranexamic acid in trauma will be assessed by the ongoing Clinical Randomisation of Antifibrinolytic in Significant Haemorrhage (CRASH) II study (www.CRASH2.LSHTM.ac.uk), in which 20 000 trauma patients worldwide are being randomized to 1 g tranexamic acid followed by a 6–8-hour infusion of a further 1 g.

Thrombosis has been the feared theoretic side effect of antifibrinolytic drugs; the Cochrane review of antifibrinolytics, however, cites studies that included over 8000 patients and demonstrated no increased risk. All antifibrinolytics are renally excreted and therefore dosage should be reduced in patients with renal failure. Because aprotinin is a bovine protein with an associated risk of anaphylaxis, a test dose must be given. After high dose aprotinin as many as 50% of patients develop specific antibodies within 3 months of exposure. An open study by Mangano et al. (2006) suggested that aprotinin usage in cardiac surgery was associated with an increased risk of myocardial infarction, stroke and renal failure. A further publication cited an increased risk of renal problems in

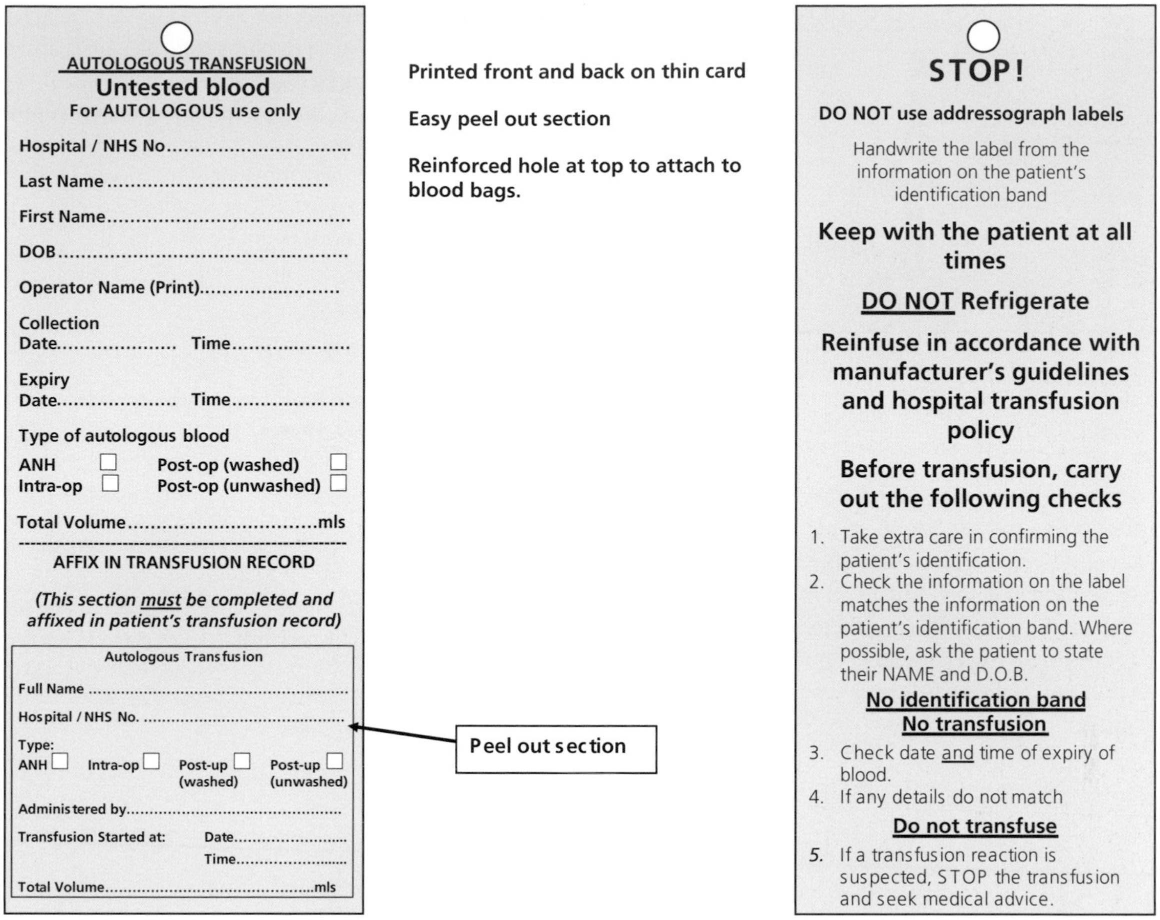

Figure 16.7 An example of an autologous blood pack label.

The following text appears in the figure:

AUTOLOGOUS TRANSFUSION
Untested blood
For AUTOLOGOUS use only

Hospital / NHS No.....................................

Last Name ....

First Name..

DOB...

Operator Name (Print).........................

Collection
Date...................... Time.....................

Expiry
Date...................... Time.....................

Type of autologous blood

ANH ☐   Post-op (washed) ☐
Intra-op ☐   Post-op (unwashed) ☐

Total Volume.................................mls

AFFIX IN TRANSFUSION RECORD

(This section must be completed and affixed in patient's transfusion record)

Autologous Transfusion

Full Name ....

Hospital / NHS No. ....

Type:
ANH ☐   Intra-op ☐   Post-up ☐   Post-up ☐
                                    (washed)   (unwashed)

Administered by..

Transfusion Started at: Date..........................
                            Time..........................

Total Volume..............................mls

Printed front and back on thin card

Easy peel out section

Reinforced hole at top to attach to blood bags.

Peel out section

STOP!

DO NOT use addressograph labels

Handwrite the label from the information on the patient's identification band

Keep with the patient at all times

DO NOT Refrigerate

Reinfuse in accordance with manufacturer's guidelines and hospital transfusion policy

Before transfusion, carry out the following checks

1. Take extra care in confirming the patient's identification.
2. Check the information on the label matches the information on the patient's identification band. Where possible, ask the patient to state their NAME and D.O.B.
   No identification band No transfusion
3. Check date and time of expiry of blood.
4. If any details do not match
   Do not transfuse
5. If a transfusion reaction is suspected, STOP the transfusion and seek medical advice.

patients receiving aprotinin compared to tranexamic acid. Blinded comparative study of aprotinin versus tranexamic acid versus ε-aminocaproic acid recruiting 3000 patients to assess safety and efficacy. Following recent publications and developments aprotinin is no longer available for use in cardiac surgery.

Desmopressin (DDAVP) is a synthetic analogue of arginine vasopressin: 1-deamino-8-D-arginine vasopressin. It releases von Willebrand factor from the endothelium and increases platelet activity. Desmopressin has been used to minimize perioperative allogeneic blood loss in cardiac surgery, but there is no convincing evidence that it does so in patients who do not have congenital bleeding disorders or uraemia.

Topical haemostatic sealants

In recent years, there has been a dramatic increase in topical haemostatic agents. Fibrin sealants and fibrin glues have been used as an adjunct to conventional methods of achieving haemostasis. The concept is to locally apply concentrated plasma derivatives to promote the conversion of fibrinogen into fibrin. The common application methods for fibrin glues include spray bottles, syringes and silastic catheters through flexible fibreoptic endoscopes.

Aside from fibrin glues, the most commonly used products are cellulose, gelatin, collagen, thrombin or aldehyde glues. The new generation topical agents are based on the concept of a fusion matrix whereby a bovine gelatin matrix is mixed with a topical thrombin solution immediately prior to use. Other new generation topical haemostatic agents include polyethylene glycol-based synthetic sealants, which have important advantages over biological substances, due to the lack of risk for transfusion-transmitted diseases. Synthetic sealants (e.g. Focalseal™) are also composed of two components, a primer and a sealant. These components are applied in two steps and then polymerized under the influence of a blue-green light from a xenon light source. Other synthetic new generation sealants consist of albumin and glutaraldehyde or hydrogels in sprayable form.

Recombinant factor VIIa

The use of recombinant factor VIIa (rFVIIa) in managing bleeding became prominent after it was used in an exsanguinating Israeli soldier with severe haemorrhage after trauma. The soldier eventually recovered. Subsequently a number of case studies and case series have described treatment with rFVIIa being beneficial in the treatment of massive coagulopathic bleeding following trauma. A recent multicentre, randomized, double-blind, placebo-controlled study examined the efficacy of rFVIIa in patients with blunt or penetrating trauma after they had received 6 units of red blood

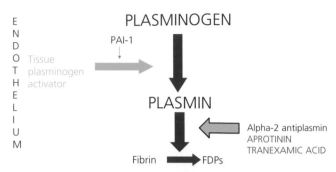

Figure 16.8 Simplified principles of fibrinolysis showing action points where aprotinin and tranexamic acid work. FDP, fibrin degradation product; PAI-1, plasminogen activator inhibitor-1.

cells, and received the first dose of their assigned medication following transfusion of a further 2 units of red blood cells (8 units in total), followed by a second and third dose, 1 and 3 hours after the initial dose. Treatment with rFVIIa in blunt trauma produced a significant reduction in transfusion requirements in patients with blunt trauma surviving for more than 48 hours, and also reduced the incidence of acute respiratory distress syndrome in all patients with blunt trauma.

The current data suggest that rFVIIa may be beneficial in uncontrolled traumatic bleeding, but it remains unclear whether the benefit is better than best practice in using blood components. rFVIIa causes localized activation of coagulation at bleeding sites, although there is an increased thrombotic risk. Since rFVIIa acts on the patient's own clotting system, adequate levels of platelets and fibrinogen are required. The required dose of rFVIIa is still under debate and as yet it is not licensed for use in reducing massive bleeding.

Further reading

A manual of blood conservation, www.transfusionguidelines.org.uk

Fergusson DA, Hébert PC, Mazer CD et al. A Comparison of Aprotinin and Lysine Analogues in High-Risk Cardiac Surgery. *New England Journal of Medicine* 2008; **358**(22): 2319–31.

Mangano DT, Tudor IC, Dietzel C et al. The risk associated with aprotonin in cardiac surgery. *New England Journal of Medicine* 2006; **354**(4): 353–65.

Munoz M, Garcia-Erce JA, Villar J, Thomas D. Blood conservation strategies in major orthopaedic surgery: efficacy, safety and European regulations. *Vox Sanguinis* 2008. DOI:10,1111/j.1423-0410.2008.01108X.

Thomas D, Thomson J, Ridler B. *A Manual for Blood Conservation*. tfm Publishing, Shrewsbury, 2005.

CHAPTER 17

Blood Substitutes and Oxygen Therapeutics

Kenneth C. Lowe

OVERVIEW

- A blood substitute has not been found. Although in widespread use, the term blood substitute, as such, should be replaced by 'red cell substitute', or, preferably, by 'oxygen therapeutic drug.'

- An ideal red cell substitute should have the same osmolarity as red cell, being able to pick up oxygen from the lungs and deliver it to the tissues. It should be free of transmissible agents, stable at room temperature for lon periods of time, non-antigenic, with no need for crossmatching and should not produce adverse immunological reactions in the recipient. It should be cheap to manufacture.

- The two approaches to developing an oxygen therapeutic are: (1) haemoglobin solutions; (2) emulsions of perfluorocarbons.

- A bovine haemoglobin solution has been approved for clinical trial, albeit only in South Africa. A few other products are at the stage where clinical trials are underway or are being planned.

Box 17.1 **Disadvantages of blood for transfusion**

- Needs human volunteer donors
- Increasingly difficult to recruit and retain donors
- Storage
- Transport
- Short shelf-life
- Potential to transmit blood-borne infectious agents
- Errors in administration may cause ABO incompatible transfusion
- Cultural and religious objections

Why is there a need for blood substitutes?

The ability to transfuse blood and blood components was one of the major medical advances of the twentieth century. Modern blood transfusion in developed countries is a universally practised and remarkably safe medical procedure. Blood or concentrated red cells are routinely transfused following extensive blood loss or as a treatment for chronic anaemia for which there is no alternative therapy. In both situations, the aim is to increase the arterial oxygen content and enhance oxygen delivery to the tissues.

In parallel with the evolution of modern transfusion medicine, there has been increasing interest in so-called 'blood or red cell substitutes'. The reason highlights some of the disadvantages of blood transfusion (Box 17.1). Blood has to be stored refrigerated (at 4°C) and transport may be a problem. The useful shelf-life of blood or red cells is only about 42 days (35 days in the UK), even with the use of modern nutrient additives, such as mannitol, glucose and adenine. Inevitably, some donated blood is wasted.

Another problem is the need to type, antibody screen and cross-match blood, due to the natural occurrence of ABO antibodies, the polymorphism of red cell membrane antigens and their immunogenicity. Despite pre-transfusion testing, immune-mediated transfusion reactions still occur due to alloimmunization to antigens on red cells, white cells, platelets and plasma proteins.

Aside from practical and physiological problems are cultural and religious objections to blood transfusion. This is best exemplified by Jehovah's Witnesses and the biblical injunction in Leviticus (17:11): 'Ye shall not eat the blood of no manner of flesh: for the life of all flesh is the blood thereof'. Jehovah's Witnesses interpret this so strictly that they refuse blood transfusions, even when their (or their child's) life is threatened.

The realization in the 1980s that human immunodeficiency virus (HIV) infection could be transmitted through the transfusion of blood products has led to increasing fear of blood donation and transfusion. This has occurred despite significant improvements in donor screening procedures and the refinement of educational policies.

All the problems outlined in Box 17.1 could, in principle, be solved by a synthetic substitute fluid with the same osmolarity as red cells that could pick up oxygen in the lungs and deliver it to the tissues. Such a blood substitute should be free of transmissible agents, stable for long periods at room temperature, non-antigenic with no need for crossmatching, and should not produce adverse immunological reactions in humans.

The search for an effective blood substitute

Arguably, the search for a blood substitute began in the mid to late nineteenth century when physicians who were frustrated by the frequent lethality caused by heterologous blood transfusion used

---

ABC of Transfusion, 4th edition, 2009. Edited by Marcela Contreras. © 2009 Blackwell Publishing, ISBN: 978-1-4051-5646-2.

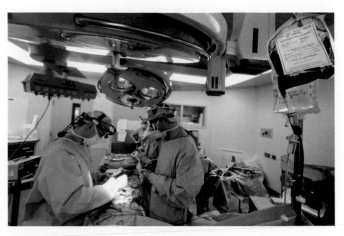

Figure 17.1 Hemopure® being used during surgery as an alternative to blood for maintaining oxygen supply to the body's vital organs. When used in this way, such products are often described as temporary oxygen therapeutic drugs. (Courtesy of Biopure Corporation, USA.)

other fluids, notably saline solutions, as alternatives. Isotonic electrolyte solutions containing gelatin or dextran are now routinely used as blood volume expanders or haemodiluents. However, such fluids have a very limited capacity to carry oxygen, due to the low solubility of the gas in aqueous systems (approximately 2–3 vol %). A blood replacement fluid capable of making a significant contribution to systemic oxygen transport could be used as an alternative to transfusing red cells. It is argued that the term 'red cell substitute' is preferred over blood substitute, since fluids currently under evaluation are primarily replacing the respiratory gas-transporting properties of erythrocytes. There is a growing use of the term 'oxygen therapeutics' in preference to blood or red cell substitutes (other terms used are antihypoxic agents and artificial oxygen carriers). Box 17.2 lists the properties required of an ideal blood substitute.

Potential blood substitutes

The two current approaches to developing blood substitutes are: (i) the development of fluids based on the naturally occurring respiratory pigment, haemoglobin, including microencapsulated haemoglobin and recombinant haemoglobin; and (ii) the use of emulsions of highly fluorinated compounds called perfluorochemicals (commonly called fluorocarbons).

Haemoglobin-based blood substitutes

Sources of haemoglobin

One major concern in the development of haemoglobin-based blood substitutes has been the source of the haemoglobin. Ideally, human haemoglobin should be used and one ready source is outdated red cells from blood banks. However, major improvements in blood storage, handling methods and stock control have resulted in reduced wastage and, consequently, less raw material.

An alternative source of haemoglobin is from slaughterhouse blood, which provides a potentially unlimited source. Hemopure® is a 13% (w/v) glutaraldehyde, cross-linked, bovine haemoglobin solution (Biopure, USA) that was licensed in South Africa as an alternative to using blood during surgery in adults (Figure 17.1). The non-human origin of the haemoglobin in Hemopure® means that it is likely to be accepted by some Jehovah's Witnesses. Importantly, this blood substitute was first approved in a country where HIV infection is common and there are serious risks of further spreading the disease

through transfusion of blood. However, in Western Europe and the USA, a bovine haemoglobin-based product may be less acceptable to patients because of concerns about possible transmission of bovine spongiform encephalopathy (BSE) infectivity.

Modified haemoglobin solutions

Early studies with the transfusion of haemoglobin solutions identified nephrotoxic effects caused by residual red cell stroma and dimers produced from the dissociation of the tetrameric haemoglobin molecule. This led to improvements in the purification and stabilizing processes for preparing haemoglobin for intravascular use.

One problem is that when released from the red cell, haemoglobin loses its ability to bind the anion 2,3-diphosphoglycerate (2,3-DPG), essential for a low oxygen affinity, as expressed by the P_{50} (i.e. partial pressure of oxygen when blood is 50% saturated). This results in high oxygen binding ($P_{50} = 15$ mmHg), with a left shift of the oxygen binding curve. One solution is to treat haemoglobin with pyridoxal-5-phosphate (pyridoxylation), an analogue of 2,3-DPG, which reduces the oxygen affinity to that of normal blood ($P_{50} = 27$ mmHg).

Unfortunately, unmodified haemoglobin dissociates into smaller fragments and is rapidly excreted through the kidneys within hours following injection. The short circulatory half-life of unmodified haemoglobin can be improved by the following:

1 Stabilizing the haemoglobin tetramer with intramolecular links (e.g. using diaspirin) to prevent dissociation.
2 Covalent coupling to a polymer, such as polyethylene glycol, producing a conjugated tetramer.
3 Polymerization with glutaraldehyde or o-raffinose forming intermolecular cross-linked haemoglobin.
4 Encapsulating pyridoxylated haemoglobin within a lipid membrane producing so-called 'synthetic red cells'.

Adverse effects of haemoglobin solutions

Nephrotoxicity

Haemoglobin solutions which are contaminated by red cell debris, free iron and haem can cause a number of adverse effects, including renal failure. This is largely overcome by current manufacturing procedures, which produce highly purified haemoglobin solutions.

Cardiovascular effects

Unfortunately, even pure haemoglobin solutions can cause adverse effects, particularly on the cardiovascular system. Hence, modified haemoglobin is desirable as a red cell substitute since the unmodified molecule produces unwanted cardiovascular effects, particularly vasoconstriction, with a marked increase in blood pressure and a fall in cardiac output. This occurs because haemoglobin tetramers extravasated from the circulation bind to nitric oxide derived from the vascular endothelium. Nitric oxide is a potent vasodilator and its removal leads to unopposed vasoconstriction.

Clinical trials and status of haemoglobin solutions

Clinical trials have been conducted with several commercial modified haemoglobin-based red cell substitutes, including o-raffinose intra- and intermolecularly cross-linked human haemoglobin (e.g. Hemolink™; Hemosol, Canada) and glutaraldehyde-polymerized human haemoglobin (e.g. PolyHeme™; Northfield, USA). However, only Hemopure® has been approved for clinical use (Figure 17.2). One newer product, Hemospan™ (Sangart, USA), contains human haemoglobin conjugated to maleimide-treated polyethylene glycol, giving a molecular mass about twice that of Hemopure®. This prevents extravasation from the circulation,

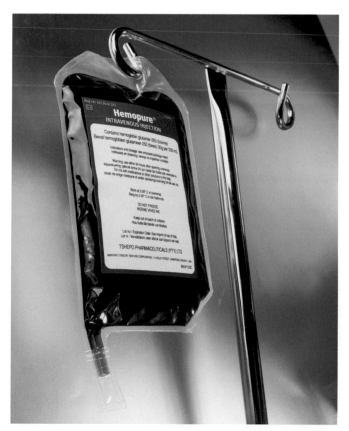

Figure 17.2 One unit of the haemoglobin-based blood substitute, Hemopure®, the first such product to be licensed for clinical use. (Courtesy of Biopure Corporation, USA.)

thereby avoiding any hypertensive side effects. Hemospan™ also has a higher affinity for oxygen (P_{50} = 5–6 mmHg) than blood and many earlier haemoglobin-based blood substitutes. The rationale is to avoid excessive oxygenation of tissues and prevent compensatory arteriolar vasoconstriction causing hypertension. This new paradigm shift in the design of blood substitutes is controversial and not without its critics. The new bovine haemoglobin-based OxyVita™ (OxyVita, USA) has similar properties.

Encapsulated haemoglobin

One way of improving the circulation time of unmodified haemoglobin is to enclose it within a lipid membrane. Haemoglobin has been encapsulated with 2,3-DPG ('neohemocytes') as the first step towards creating synthetic red blood cells. If the haemoglobin is treated with pyridoxal-5-phosphate, a stable product is produced. Encapsulation prevents renal clearance of haemoglobin. Additionally, enzymes, such as superoxide dismutase and catalase, can be incorporated into the liposomes to scavenge potentially damaging oxygen radicals.

Human recombinant haemoglobin

Human haemoglobin has been synthesized by genetically modified bacteria, yeast or plants (so-called 'cell factories'). Such recombinant haemoglobins (rHbs) have oxygen binding properties similar to normal human haemoglobin. This approach avoids using human or animal blood as raw material, thereby overcoming the problem of transmitting infectious agents. In a first-generation rHb – rHb1.1, known as Optro™ (Baxter, USA) – some amino acid sequences were replaced to prevent molecular dissociation and giving acceptable oxygen binding characteristics. A new European project, Genomics and Blood Substitutes for 21st Century Europe (acronym EuroBloodSubstitutes), is developing a technological baseline for producing novel haem proteins and blood substitute components using microorganisms.

Recombinant haemoglobins are an exciting way forward for blood substitutes since 'tailor-made' molecules can, in principle, be produced. Recombinant technology is being used to produce haemoglobin mutants with altered affinity for nitric oxide, thereby overcoming the transient, hypertensive side effects considered previously as a flaw in the usefulness of haemoglobin red cell substitutes. It is not yet clear whether this type of haemoglobin can be produced in a larger scale at lower cost. Box 17.3 details the advantages of rHb.

Perfluorochemical emulsions

Perfluorochemicals are organic compounds in which hydrogen atoms have been replaced with fluorine. They are clear, odourless, inert fluids, which are radiopaque. The compounds are extremely

---

Box 17.3 **Advantages of recombinant haemoglobin**

- Virus free
- No residual stromal contamination
- Unconstrained supply
- Can be engineered for specific requirements

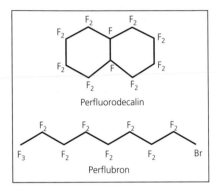

Figure 17.3 Chemical structures of two perfluorochemicals. Both the cyclic (perfluorodecalin) and linear (perflubron) compounds have been tested as red cell substitutes in humans.

unreactive chemically, due to the strength of the carbon–fluorine bonds (Box 17.4).

Perfluorochemical liquids dissolve large volumes of respiratory gases (up to 45 vol % oxygen per atmosphere at 37°C) and the relationship between oxygen tension and partial pressure is linear. This contrasts with the characteristic sigmoid curve of whole blood (and haemoglobin). Because perfluorochemical liquids are immiscible with blood and water, they must be emulsified before intravascular use. The target droplet size is about 0.2 μm. Following intravascular injection, emulsion droplets are removed from the circulation and temporarily stored in phagocytic cells of the monocyte–macrophage (reticuloendothelial) system. Eventually, the perfluorochemicals are excreted from the body by exhalation.

Since the late 1970s, several emulsions, containing one or more perfluorochemicals (Figure 17.3), have been developed as potential oxygen therapeutics. The first emulsion produced commercially was Fluosol®, a 20% (w/v) formulation containing two fluorocarbons, perfluorodecalin and perfluorotripropylamine (Green Cross Corporation, Japan). A similar perfluorocarbon-based oxygen carrier, Perftoran (Perftoran, Russia), was approved in Russia in 1996 for use in severe anaemia, haemorrhagic shock and cardiac surgery. Perftoran has been used in over 2000 patients, but little information on its use is available.

Fluosol® was the first perfluorochemical emulsion evaluated as a blood substitute/oxygen therapeutic in humans and extensive clinical trials were reported in the 1980s. It was approved (in 1990) by the American Food and Drug Administration Committee for use in restricted doses and in high risk patients, for oxygenating the distal coronary vascular bed during balloon angioplasty. However, in 1994, Green Cross ceased manufacturing Fluosol® due to the lack of interest from physicians and poor sales in their angioplasty indication. Improvements in angioplasty technology had made the need for Fluosol® redundant.

Fluosol® is now regarded as a first generation fluorocarbon emulsion and the experience gained from its clinical use informed the development of improved emulsions, involving:

- the production of more concentrated emulsions, which, in principle, can carry more oxygen
- marked improvements in emulsion stability at room temperature, thus giving acceptable shelf-lives.

The current front runner amongst the second generation, concentrated fluorocarbon emulsions is Oxygent™, produced by the Alliance Pharmaceutical Corporation, San Diego. Oxygent™ is a 60% (w/v) emulsion of perflubron with 4% (w/v) egg yolk phospholipids as surfactant. Oxygent™ is stable for up to 1 year at room temperature and is rapidly eliminated from the body, with a half-time of about 4 days.

Oxygent™ has been tested in over 1300 patients. The infusion of perflubron emulsion into patients breathing oxygen was found to be more effective than autologous blood or colloid solution in maintaining cardiovascular function and tissue oxygen supply. In 500 general surgery patients, treatment with Oxygent™ reduced the frequency and volume of blood used. In 2001, Alliance suspended enrolment in a phase III cardiac surgery study with Oxygent™ to evaluate an increased incidence of stroke in patients. New licensing, development and marketing agreements with pharmaceutical companies in China, Europe and Canada are being persued for the clinical and regulatory development of the drug for organ protection against hypoxia during surgery.

Conclusion

This chapter reviews potential blood substitutes or oxygen therapeutic drugs. A bovine haemoglobin-based product has been approved for clinical use, albeit in a country where blood-borne disease is endemic. The development of other haemoglobin- and perfluorochemical-based materials has progressed to the stage where advanced clinical trials are underway or planned.

Blood substitutes seem to have a definite role in surgery to avoid and minimize blood transfusions. The avoidance of allogeneic blood would be beneficial to the patient and help the transfusion services conserve blood. This is a dynamic and forward-looking area of biotechnology. It is anticipated that products will emerge that will be useful, not only as intravascular gas carriers in transfusion medicine, but as biopharmaceuticals for other biomedical disciplines.

Further reading

Winslow RM, ed. *Blood Substitutes*. Academic Press, London, 2006.
Natanson C, Kern SJ, Lurie P et al. *JAMA* 2008; **299**(17): 2304–12.

CHAPTER 18

Appropriate Use of Blood and Better Blood Transfusion

Mike Murphy

OVERVIEW

- The promotion of safe and appropriate use of blood is part of clinical governance in hospitals.
- Education and training programmes for doctors should emphasize the appropriate use of blood.
- Clinical research is essential to provide an adequate evidence base for transfusion and the use of alternatives to transfusion.
- New approaches to the prevention of 'wrong' blood transfusion should be considered including the use of automated bedside systems with barcode patient identification.
- Data on blood usage should be provided to clinical teams so they can compare their practice with others.
- Hospitals should improve information systems to facilitate routine monitoring of blood usage.
- Collaboration within clinical teams and between hospitals is essential to promote good transfusion practice.
- Better Blood Transfusion recommendations should have a high priority in hospitals in terms of patient safety and ensuring best use of a scarce resource.
- There is potential for reducing the use of fresh frozen plasma and platelet transfusions, and for further reductions in the use of red cell transfusions.
- Renewed efforts should be made to reduce blood usage in medical patients.
- The identification and management of preoperative anaemia avoids the need for perioperative red cell transfusion.
- Better use should be made of alternatives to transfusion in surgical patients.
- Good communication is essential between clinicians and blood bank staff about the timely and effective use of blood in patients with massive bleeding.
- The decision to use recombinant activated factor VII in a patient with uncontrolled bleeding must be made by individual clinicians guided by hospital policies and advice from haematologists with expertise in transfusion medicine.

- Advances in information technology could be used to provide 'decision support' for doctors considering transfusion in individual patients.
- Patients should be better educated to exercise choice about blood transfusion and the use of alternatives to transfusion.

Although the quality and safety of blood in the UK is amongst the best in the world, blood transfusion is not free from risk. The most logical approach to reducing the risk of transfusion is only to use blood when it is strictly clinically necessary and there is no alternative.

There has been a recent focus on better blood transfusion practice worldwide because of concerns about patient safety, documented variations in blood usage, and increasing costs of transfusion. In the UK, this work has been termed the Better Blood Transfusion initiative. This chapter will review what activities have taken place to improve the use of blood and to promote alternatives to transfusion.

History of the Better Blood Transfusion initiative in the UK

The Health Service Circular (HSC) 1998/224 *Better Blood Transfusion* detailed the action required of hospitals and clinicians to improve transfusion practice. Its recommendations were based on presentations and workshops in a symposium on evidence-based blood transfusion held by the UK Chief Medical Officers (CMOs) in London in July 1998. A survey in 2001 of the implementation of these initial Better Blood Transfusion recommendations showed that most hospitals had established hospital transfusion committees (HTCs), were participating in the Serious Hazards of Transfusion (SHOT) scheme, and had protocols for the administration of blood (Table 18.1). However, there was evidence of poor training of clinical staff, few protocols for the appropriate use of blood and audits of transfusion practice, and limited use of autologous transfusion.

A second UK CMOs' seminar on blood transfusion was held in October 2001, focusing on avoiding unnecessary transfusion. The HSC 2002/009 *Better Blood Transfusion: appropriate use of blood* was issued in July 2002, detailing the further actions required of hospitals, the National Blood Service (NBS) and clinicians to improve transfusion practice. Hospitals were required to develop hospital transfusion teams comprising a lead consultant for transfusion,

ABC of Transfusion, 4th edition, 2009. Edited by Marcela Contreras. © 2009 Blackwell Publishing, ISBN: 978-1-4051-5646-2.

Table 18.1 Progress on the implementation of Better Blood Transfusion strategies since 2001.

	2001	2003	2004	2006
Hospitals completing the questionnaire survey	220/320 (69%)	122/259 (47%)	160/169 (95%)	156/173 (90%)
Participation in SHOT scheme	96%	100%	99%	95%
Hospitals with a HTC	91%	98%	99%	97%
% staff trained as:				
Phlebotomists	79%	97%	97%	74%
Porters	47%	75%	80%	69%
Nurses	78%	52%	73%	83%
Medical staff	34%	53%	60%	87%
Transfusion practitioner in post	14%	50%	68%	92%
Lead consultant in post	–	74%	83%	90%
Protocol for the transfusion process	98%	97%	98%	96%
Protocols for the use of blood:				
Surgical blood ordering schedule	67%	87%	92%	97%
Red cell transfusion*	34%	44% (critical care) 34% (surgical)	46% (critical care) 39% (surgical)	70% (critical care) 58% (surgical)

HTC, hospital transfusion committee; SHOT, Serious Hazards of Transfusion.

* The question about red cell transfusion protocols was different between the 2001 and the later surveys. In 2001, the question asked if the hospital had a general red cell transfusion protocol. In 2003 and 2005, the question referred to specific protocols for critical care and surgical patients.

a specialist practitioner of transfusion (usually, but not necessarily, a specialist nurse) and a senior biomedical scientist in transfusion. The role of the hospital transfusion team is to promote good transfusion practice by implementing actions approved by the HTC, which has the overall remit for improving hospital transfusion practice, and to be a resource for training all hospital staff involved in blood transfusion, primarily facilitated by specialist practitioners of transfusion.

A CMOs' National Blood Transfusion Committee and 12 regional transfusion committees were established in England in 2001 with a primary remit to support the Better Blood Transfusion initiative.

The results of further surveys in 2003 and 2004 indicated some progress in the implementation of Better Blood Transfusion initiatives, including training, and the number of hospitals with transfusion practitioners (see Table 18.1). However, the results also indicated the need for further progress in the training of some staff groups, particularly nurses and doctors, the development of hospital transfusion teams and protocols for the appropriate use of blood, the provision of information to patients, and the use of perioperative cell salvage.

Evidence base for the appropriate use of blood and alternatives to transfusion

Recent high quality evidence in the form of systematic reviews of the literature and well conducted clinical trials has disproved some widely accepted indications for transfusion, and has had a major impact on changing transfusion practice. Examples include:

1 A randomized clinical trial of a restrictive red cell transfusion strategy (red cells transfused if the haemoglobin concentration fell below 7 g/dl) was at least as effective and possibly superior to a liberal transfusion strategy (red cells transfused if the haemoglobin fell below 10 g/dl) in critically ill patients.

2 A systematic review of 57 trials of fresh frozen plasma (FFP) found that only three were of adequate design and power, and two showed no clinical benefit of the use of FFP.

3 A systematic review of alternatives to transfusion found that only the use of antifibrinolytic drugs, such as aprotinin and tranexamic acid, and perioperative cell salvage consistently reduced the use of donor blood.

Audit as a tool to improve transfusion practice

Sequential national audits by the NBS and Royal College of Physicians have shown improvements in transfusion practice with fewer patients not wearing a wristband (6% in 2005 versus 10% in 2003) and fewer at risk from lack of observations (34% with no observations in the first 30 minutes of transfusion in 2005, compared with 47% in 2003). However, there is still substantial evidence of transfused patients being put at risk of 'wrong' transfusions because of poor patient identification (Figure 18.1) and inadequate monitoring during transfusion.

There is evidence of wide variation between hospitals in the use of blood for common surgical procedures. A recent audit in primary hip replacement surgery in the Oxford hospitals showed a range of 23–58% in the proportion of patients who were transfused. The majority of patients who were transfused only received 1 or 2 units of blood and most of these were discharged with a haemoglobin above 10 g/dl. If they had not been transfused, they would still have

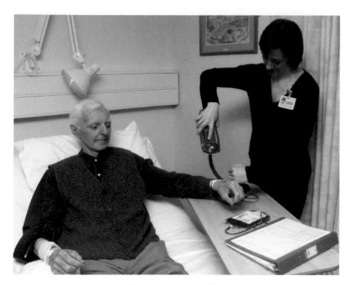

Figure 18.1 Poor patient identification should be avoided with the use of a handheld computer and barcode patient identification for safe bedside transfusion. (Reproduced with permission from the front cover of the September 2003 edition of *Transfusion*)

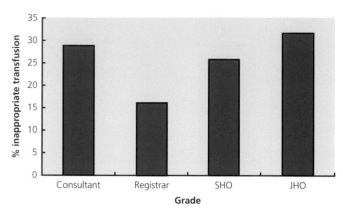

Figure 18.3 The percentage of inappropriate transfusions with different grades of medical staff in an audit of red cell transfusions in Northern Ireland. JHO, junior house officer; SHO, senior house officer. (With permission of the Northern Ireland Regional Transfusion Committee.)

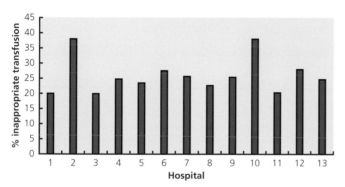

Figure 18.2 The percentage of inappropriate transfusions in an audit of red cell transfusions in 13 hospitals in Northern Ireland. (With permission of the Northern Ireland Regional Transfusion Committee.)

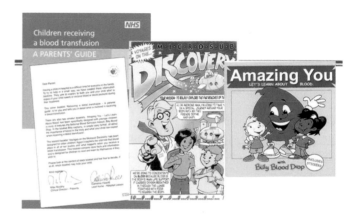

Figure 18.4 Examples of patient information leaflets.

had a haemoglobin above 8 g/dl, which would not be expected to impair postoperative recovery.

A recent audit in Northern Ireland estimated that 20% of red cell transfusions were inappropriate. This proportion of inappropriate transfusions was similar in all 13 hospitals surveyed (Figure 18.2), and was not influenced by clinical specialty or grade of doctor requesting the transfusion (Figure 18.3). Repeated rounds of comparative audit, where data from individual hospitals or clinical specialties are readily compared with others, has been shown to be a powerful tool for improving practice in other areas of medicine such as myocardial infarction and stroke.

Better Blood Transfusion activities

Examples of Better Blood Transfusion initiatives
Specific initiatives in the UK have included the following:
1 Advice to hospitals on how to implement Better Blood Transfusion strategies, including the resources required, in the form of a 'toolkit' (available on www.transfusionguidelines.org.uk).

A summary of the indications for the use of blood is also provided (see Chapter 4).
2 The production of national patient information leaflets for adults, children and parents (Figure 18.4).
3 The development of national and local contingency plans for blood shortages, highlighting the need for each hospital to plan for acute and chronic blood shortages and to reduce blood usage as an important priority.
4 More support from the NBS, specifically the development of its hospital liaison function, comprising a transfusion liaison nurse, a hospital liaison manager and a joint medical consultant in each region to support specialist transfusion practitioners, blood transfusion laboratory scientific staff and clinicians in hospitals.

Review of progress since 2002
Results of questionnaire surveys in 2003 and 2004 indicate progress since 2001 in the proportion of hospitals with HTCs, the training of some staff groups, the number of hospitals with transfusion practitioners, and the development of protocols for the use of blood (see Table 18.1). However, the results also indicated that further progress is needed.

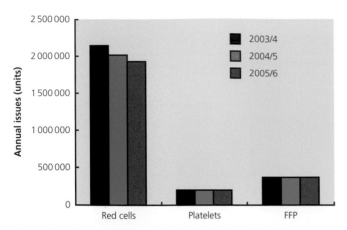

Figure 18.5 Change in the issues of red cell, platelet and fresh frozen plasma (FFP) units in England from 2003/4 to 2005/6.

Effect on blood usage

As a result of these efforts to use blood more appropriately and possibly because of other factors, such as increases in the cost of blood, the use of red cell transfusions in England fell by 5.7% in 2004/5, and by a further 4.4% in 2005/6 (Figure 18.5). The use of FFP and platelet concentrates has changed very little.

Where does blood go?

Red cell transfusions are most commonly used in medicine for patients with cancer or gastrointestinal bleeding, and in surgery for cardiac and orthopaedic procedures. Medical use now accounts for about 65% of red cell usage (for many years, medical and surgical use were both approximately 50%). Most of the recent reduction in red cell usage has occurred in surgery.

Strategies for reducing blood use in surgical patients

There is a varied emphasis on blood management by clinical teams. Some teams carry out major procedures by attention to patient care throughout the perioperative period, resulting in avoidance of transfusion (Box 18.1; see also Chapter 16).

After the introduction of guidelines in one large hospital in Scotland, data on blood use in relation to haemoglobin before and after transfusion were fed back to clinical teams with suggestions about appropriate blood use. Audits were carried out before the initiative and after 1 year; red cell use decreased by 20% with no demonstrable effect on morbidity or mortality.

Strategies for reducing blood use in medical patients

Good blood management depends on many of the same principles as have been described for surgical patients, including the identification of the cause of anaemia and its appropriate investigation and treatment, the timely estimation of blood counts and haemostasis in massive blood loss, and the implementation of local policies for blood use with education and audit (Box 18.2).

Recombinant erythropoietin improves the quality of life of patients with chronic renal failure by the effective treatment of

---

Box 18.1 Strategies for reducing blood use in surgical patients

Preoperative
• Establishment of preoperative assessment clinics
• Identification and correction of anaemia
• Avoidance of drugs interfering with haemostasis, e.g. anticoagulants, or drugs with antiplatelet activity for a period of time prior to surgery

Operative
• Good anaesthetic and surgical technique
• Avoidance of hypothermia
• Reduction of regional vascular pressure
• Cell salvage
• Point-of-care testing (for blood count and haemostasis) to guide the use of blood components
• Use of antifibrinolytic drugs such as aprotinin and tranexamic acid

Postoperative
• Implementation of local guidelines for the use of blood, based on national guidelines, with education, audit and feedback of data to clinical teams
• Minimizing the volume of blood collected for laboratory samples
• Cell salvage

Box 18.2 Strategies for reducing blood use in medical patients

• Identification and correction of anaemia with appropriate haematinics
• Use of recombinant erythropoietin for patients with anaemia due to chronic renal failure and some cancers
• Timely estimation of blood counts and haemostasis in massive blood loss
• Implementation of local guidelines for the use of blood with education, audit and feedback of data to clinical teams

---

anaemia. It is also effective in the avoidance of blood transfusion in some cancer patients.

Management of massive blood loss

The usual presentation is as an emergency in accident and emergency, obstetrics or surgery. The restoration of an adequate circulating volume is the most important immediate aim, followed by treatment of any surgical source of bleeding and the correction of haemostatic abnormalities with blood components.

Recombinant activated factor VII appears to be effective in the treatment of severe haemorrhage unresponsive to standard management, but as yet there are few data on its safety and effectiveness.

Future prospects for the Better Blood Transfusion initiative

There has been better recent recognition of the risks of transfusion and the safety of restrictive transfusion policies. Although blood usage is reducing, recent audit data continue to provide evidence of high levels of inappropriate use. Better education about good transfusion practice, wider adoption of algorithms for blood management including alternatives to transfusion where relevant, and the adoption of conservative transfusion thresholds should result in further reductions in blood usage without compromising patient safety. The Better Blood Transfusion initiative has been relaunched in 2007, following a further survey in 2006 of the implementation of the recommendations in the HSC 2002/009 (see Table 18.1), with a third UK CMOs' seminar and the issue of HSC 2007/001 *Better Blood Transfusion: safe and appropriate use of blood.*

Further reading

Carless PA, Henry DA, Moxey AJ, O'Connell DL, Brown T, Fergusson DA. Cell salvage for minimising perioperative allogeneic blood transfusion. *Cochrane Database of Systematic Reviews* 2006, Issue 4. Art. No. CD001888.

Hebert PC, Wells G, Blajchman MA, et al. A multicenter, randomized, controlled trial of transfusion requirements in critical care. *New England Journal of Medicine* 2004; **340**: 409–17.

Henry DA, Moxley AJ, Carless PA, et al. Anti-fibrinolytic use for minimising perioperative allogeneic blood transfusion. *Cochrane Database of Systematic Reviews* 2007, Issue 4. Art. No. CD001886.

Murphy MF, Howell C. Survey of the implementation of the recommendations in the Health Service Circular 2002/009 'Better Blood Transfusion'. *Transfusion Medicine* 2005; **15**: 453–60.

Stansworth SJ, Birchall J, Doree CJ, Hyde C. Recombinant factor VIIa for the prevention and treatment of bleeding in patients without haemophilia. *Cochrane Database Systematic Reviews* 2007; **18**(2): CD005011.

Stanworth SJ, Brunskill SJ, Hyde CJ, McClelland DBL, Murphy MF. What is the evidence base for the clinical use of FFP: a systematic review of randomised controlled trials. British Journal of Haematology 2004; **126**: 139–52.

References

Department of Health. *Better Blood Transfusion: appropriate use of blood.* HSC 2002/009. Department of Health, London, 2002.

Department of Health. *Better Blood Transfusion: safe and appropriate use of blood.* HSC 2007/001. Department of Health, London, 2007.

CHAPTER 19

Stem Cell Transplantation and Cellular Therapies

Aleksandar Mijovic, Derwood Pamphilon and Suzanne Watt

OVERVIEW

- Haemopoietic stem cell (HSC) transplantation is currently the sole curative option for several haematological disorders. A paradigm shift from eradication of host cells to manipulation of immune mechanisms, in view of exploiting the antitumour potential of the graft, has occurred.

- Peripheral blood has largely replaced bone marrow as the source of HSCs; donor availability has been greatly improved by the establishment of volunteer donor panels, which currently have over 10 million donors worldwide.

- Umbilical cord blood is a suitable source of allogeneic HSCs. It is universally available, poses no risk to the donor and is associated with a lower incidence of graft-versus-host disease (GvHD), allowing the use of cells with up to two major human leucocyte antigen (HLA)–antigen mismatches.

- Therapies using specific cell subsets allow selective antitumour effects (cytotoxic T-lymphocytes, natural killer cells) or dampening of GvHD and autoimmununity (mesenchymal cells, T-regulatory cells).

- Bone marrow, fetal or cord blood stem cells can undergo differentiation into neural, cardiac muscle, liver, epithelial and skin cells. Stem cell-based therapies are likely to be used in the future for conditions such as Parkinson's disease, diabetes, arthritis, multiple sclerosis and cardiovascular diseases.

Haemopoietic stem cell transplantation

Haemopoietic stem cell (HSC) transplantation is currently the main therapeutic, and often the sole curative option for a variety of haematological disorders (Table 19.1). The original concept of allogeneic stem cell transplantation implied eradication of host myeloid and lymphoid cells by use of high dose cytotoxic drugs and/or radiation ('conditioning') prior to the infusion of the donor's haemopoietic cells. Although toxic, complete ablation of the host haemopoietic and immune system was considered essential for disease cure and to minimize the risk of graft rejection. The donor's immune reaction against the host, graft-versus-host

ABC of Transfusion, 4th edition, 2009. Edited by Marcela Contreras. © 2009 Blackwell Publishing, ISBN: 978-1-4051-5646-2.

Table 19.1 'Standard of care' indications for haemopoietic stem cell transplantation (modified from the European Group for Blood and Marrow Transplantation 2005).

Allogeneic
Acute myeloid leukaemia: high risk/relapsed
Acute lymphoblastic leukaemia: high risk/relapsed
Chronic myeloid leukaemia
Myelodysplastic syndromes
Aplastic anaemia
Thalassemia major
Primary immune deficiencies

Autologous
Acute myeloid leukaemia: high risk/relapsed
Non-Hodgkin's lymphoma, high grade/relapsed
Hodgkin's disease: relapsed
Multiple myeloma
Germ cell cancer: relapsed
Ewing's sarcoma: high risk/relapsed

Table 19.2 Principles of non-myeloablative (reduced intensity) conditioning transplantation.

- Strong immunosuppressive effect (fludarabine, campath 1H, antilymphocyte globulin) to prevent rejection
- Reduced myelosuppression and organ toxicity
- Minimise graft versus host disease by establishing mixed chimerism
- Convert to full donor chimerism by tapering post-transplant immunosuppresion and addition of donor lymphocyte infusions

disease (GvHD), complicates allogeneic HSC transplantation and is one of the main causes of morbidity and mortality. However, advances in transplantation immunology, coupled with clinical data, have highlighted the role of donor immune cells in establishing engraftment and preventing disease recurrence via the graft-versus-tumour effect. The delicate balance between the beneficial and harmful immunological effects of the graft became the field of intense research, from which ensued the concept of non-myeloablative HSC transplantation (Table 19.2).

Autologous HSC transplantation, where the donor and the recipient are the same person, stemmed from the concept of chemotherapy intensification ('more is better'). Since more

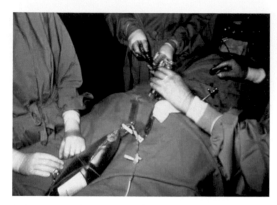

Figure 19.1 Harvesting bone marrow from the posterior iliac crest.

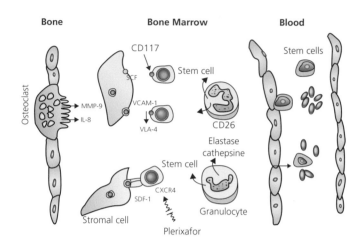

Figure 19.2 Mechanisms of haemopoietic stem cell mobilization. AMD3100, CXCR4 antagonist; CD26, serine-type proteinase; CD117, SCF receptor; CXCR4, chemokine receptor 4, ligand for SDF-1; IL-8, interleukin 8; MMP-9, metalloproteinase 9; SCF, stem cell factor; SDF-1, stroma-derived factor 1; VCAM-1, vascular cell adhesion molecule 1 (CD106); VLA-4, integrin, ligand of VCAM-1.

Table 19.3 Pros and cons of peripheral blood stem cell transplantation compared with bone marrow transplantation.

Pros
Higher CD34+ cell counts
Faster neutrophil and platelet recovery
Convenience of collection
Lower costs compared to bone marrow harvesting
No admission to hospital; no general anaesthesia

Cons
Use of mobilizing agents
Venous access may be a problem
Higher risk of chronic graft versus host disease

Questionable
Improvement of survival

chemotherapy causes unacceptable bone marrow toxicity, HSCs can be collected prior to, and infused after, intensive chemo/radiotherapy in order to rescue the patient. In this setting, immunological disparity is not an issue, but reinfusion of malignant cells remains contentious. Gene marking experiments have shown that relapse may originate from the autologous graft, not just from the residual cells in the body that survive cytotoxic therapy. Various chemical and immunological methods of cleansing the graft of tumour cells ('purging') exist, but their clinical benefits are still unclear.

For years, the only source of HSC was the bone marrow, obtained by needle aspiration from the posterior iliac crest under general anaesthesia (Figure 19.1). Bone marrow harvest is a low risk procedure, though serious adverse events have occurred; the procedure requires admission to hospital for 1–2 days and causes discomfort for about a week.

By 1990 it was established that HSCs can be 'mobilized' from bone marrow into the blood by chemotherapy and haemopoietic growth factors (e.g. granulocyte and granulocyte-macrophage colony-stimulating factor (G-CSF and GM-CSF, respectively). HSC mobilization is a complex process involving several adhesion molecules that hold HSC in close contact with the bone marrow stroma (Figure 19.2). When the stem cells are released into the circulation, they can be collected by cytapheresis, using cell separators. Peripheral blood-derived HSC (PBSC) quickly became the preferred source of HSC: in 2003, 97% of autologous transplants and 65% of allogeneic transplants in Europe were derived from peripheral blood. This change was due to faster neutrophil and platelet regeneration, but also to the convenience of collection (Table 19.3). Problems of PBSC collection include poor venous access, which occasionally requires the placement of a venous catheter, and the need to administer a mobilizing agent. Patients often have a combination of chemotherapy and a haemopoietic growth factor (nearly always G-CSF), but donors can only be given G-CSF. The drug has few serious side effects, although it commonly causes bone pain, headache and fatigue. Fears that G-CSF might stimulate dormant leukaemic clones have not materialized so far. The new mobilizing agent (AMD3100) targets specific mobilization mechanisms and holds much promise for the future (Figure 19.2). Finally, unless depleted of T lymphocytes, PBSC transplantation increases the risk of chronic GvHD.

Numerous studies have demonstrated the correlation between the speed of haematological regeneration after HSC transplantation and the cell dose infused. CD34, a sialomucin present on immature haemopoietic cells, is a surrogate marker for stem cells. At least 2×10^6/kg, and preferably 5×10^6/kg, CD34+ cells are required to achieve neutrophil and platelet regeneration within 10–14 days after autologous PBSC transplantation (Figure 19.3). In allogeneic transplantation, less than 2×10^6/kg CD34+ cells are associated with higher transplant-related mortality. Most transplant centres require 4×10^6/kg CD34+ cells for allogeneic transplants.

Limited availability of human leucocyte antigen (HLA) matched siblings prompted the search for alternative donors. Volunteer, unrelated donor panels rapidly grew, reaching over 10 million donors worldwide in 2006. As a result, donor availability increased from 25–40% to 70–80%. However, recruitment, running costs, bone marrow/PBSC harvesting and shipment have added to the overall costs of HSC transplantation.

In the mid-1990s umbilical cord blood emerged as a suitable source of allogeneic HSCs (Figure 19.4). Cord blood can be

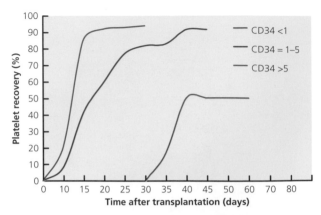

Figure 19.3 Correlation of CD34+ cell dose in HSC harvest with the platelet recovery after autologous transplantation. CD34+ cell dose is given as millions per kg body weight.

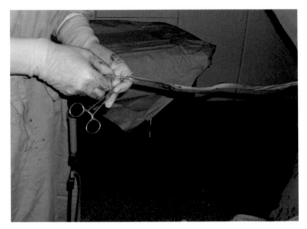

Figure 19.4 Cord blood collection with the placenta *in utero*. (Courtesy of Dr S. Querol.)

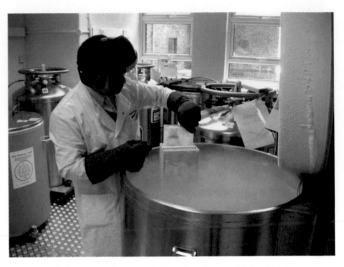

Figure 19.5 Storage of haemopoietic cells in tanks with liquid nitrogen.

collected from siblings for specific patients, or from volunteer donors for unrelated patients. Cord blood is universally available in donor registries, poses no risk to the donor, and facilitates recruitment of ethnic minority donors. It is also virtually free of latent viruses (e.g. cytomegalovirus (CMV), Epstein–Barr virus (EBV)), and is associated with a lower incidence of GvHD, allowing the use of cord blood cells with up to two major HLA–antigen mismatches. However, because of low absolute stem cell counts and consequently delayed haematological and immune regeneration, use of cord blood remained largely restricted to paediatric patients. In recent years, double cord blood transplantation and other transplant modalities circumvented the problem of the low stem cell dose in adults, and ex *vivo* cell expansion may widen the scope of cord blood transplantation further. Over 6000 cord blood transplants had been carried out worldwide by the end of 2006 and the results are encouraging.

HSCs may be given 'fresh', ideally up to 48 hours after collection. Whereas this is the norm in the allogeneic setting, fresh cells are rarely used for autologous transplants because of limited conditioning options. Cryopreservation allows storage of HSCs, which remain viable and capable of marrow repopulation for an

undetermined time, but certainly for 5–10 years, if kept under adequate storage conditions. Although storage at –80°C for about 6 months does not affect function, most centres store HSCs at temperatures below –130°C in the vapour phase of liquid nitrogen (Figure 19.5). To minimize dehydration and ice formation during freezing, cells are frozen at a controlled rate, in the presence of cryoprotectants such as dimethyl-sulphoxide. When required for infusion into the patient, cells are rapidly thawed at 37°C and immediately infused.

The HSC product may need to be further manipulated to remove or select some of the cellular components. Prior to freezing, bone marrow or cord blood is processed to the mononuclear cell fraction, which contains the stem cells. In addition to volume reduction, this removes the red cells and most of the plasma and can therefore be used in the setting of ABO incompatibility. In an attempt to prevent GvHD, peripheral blood or bone marrow can be T lymphocyte-depleted. Though the role of T cell depletion is controversial, several methods based on 'negative selection' exist: T cell rosetting, monoclonal antibodies, immunotoxins, etc. In addition, positive CD34+ cell selection by antibodies coupled to magnetic particles is used for T cell depletion, and to provide stem cells for *ex vivo* expansion.

Because of the increase in the demand and diversity of cellular products, the development of quality assurance systems became essential to guarantee the safety and quality of the product and service. Within the framework of the EU Directive on Tissues and Cells, and the Code of Practice for Tissue Banks and the Human Tissue Act in the UK, establishments that collect, process and store human stem cells have to be licensed or accredited for this function. Regulatory acts concern all parts of the process (Table 19.4).

Cellular therapies

Immunotherapy

Doctors and scientists have developed a number of ways to direct immune cells or antibodies to recognize and eliminate cancer or

Table 19.4 Components of quality assurance (modified from the Department of Health Code of Practice for Tissue Banks).

- Facilities (buildings, environment, materials, equipment)
- Personnel, responsibilities and training
- Donor selection
- Control of tissues, materials and services (contracts/agreements, storage, traceability)
- Process control (validation, release and discard of tissues, audits, complaints, non-conformance)
- Finished product control (packaging, labelling, transport)
- Documentation (standard operating procedures, specifications, records)

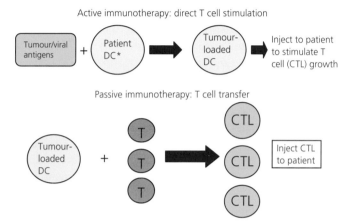

Figure 19.6 Active and passive cellular immunotherapy. CTL, cytotoxic T lymphocyte; DC, dendritic cell.

virus-infected cells. Immunotherapy may be divided as follows (Figure 19.6):

1 *Active immunotherapy*: the patient's own immune responses are stimulated, for example by vaccination with dendritic cells that present tumour antigens or DNA.

2 *Passive immunotherapy*: immunity is provided by the transfer of lymphocytes (cellular immunotherapy) or antibodies (humoral immunotherapy) with antitumour reactivity. Lymphocytes may be activated *in vitro* by dendritic cells that stimulate antitumour responses.

In the treatment of leukaemia, doctors first tried to stimulate the patients' own anticancer immunity by immunizing them with leukaemic blast cells during remission. In the setting of allogeneic stem cell transplantation, dramatic responses were described 16 years ago in three patients with chronic myeloid leukaemia (CML) who had relapsed after transplant but who achieved remission when lymphocytes from the bone marrow donor were transfused to them. All three patients were alive 13 years later as the result of the graft-versus-leukaemia (GvL) effect. Subsequently it was shown that these donor leucocyte infusions were effective in 75% of CML patients. The response rate in patients with acute myeloid and lymphoblastic leukaemia (AML and ALL, respectively) is much lower (less than 25%). HSC transplant patients are also vulnerable to infections with CMV, EBV and adenovirus and impressive antiviral responses have been recorded after the infusion of virus-specific donor T lymphocytes in the post-transplant period.

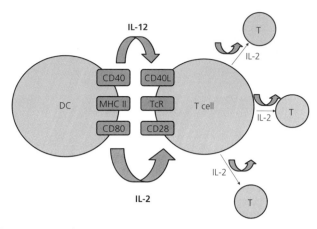

Figure 19.7 Dendritic and T cells interact via cell surface ligands. Tumour or viral antigens are presented to the T cell receptor (TcR) in association with the major histocompatibility complex (MHC) II. Dendritic cells (DC) produce interleukin-12 (IL-12) and both the dendritic and T cells secrete interleukin-2 (IL-2), leading to T cell activation.

In patients with solid tumours, the principal approach has been to immunize them with autologous tumour-loaded dendritic cells, which then present the tumour antigens to their T cells. This causes them to become cytotoxic to tumour cells; they are then called cytotoxic T lymphocytes (CTLs).

T lymphocytes

One of the reasons that leukaemia and other cancers develop is that they appear to be poorly recognized by the body's immune system. Tumour cells must display antigens like CD80 (Figure 19.7) and CD54 – an important adhesion molecule – which are involved in immune recognition so that effector cells (e.g. T lymphocytes, natural killer (NK) cells) are able to kill them. In some cancers, such as acute lymphoblastic leukaemia, these antigens are downregulated, helping the tumour cells to avoid detection.

Dendritic cells process tumour-derived peptides and present them bound to HLA antigens on their surface to activate the T cells via the T cell receptor (TcR). A second or co-stimulatory signal is given by the binding of CD80 and CD40 on dendritic cells with CD28 and CD40 ligand on T cells. This results in the production of lymphokines such as interleukin (IL) 12 and IL-2. T cells undergo expansion and may then recognize tumour cells as foreign. This is known as the major histocompatibility complex (MHC) restricted response. If one of the co-stimulatory signals is missing then a state of tolerance develops (Figure 19.7).

Natural killer cells

Natural killer cells are able to recognize tumour and virally infected cells. They lack the TcR but express other receptors, such as the inhibitory killer immunoglobulin-like receptors (KIRs) which bind to HLA class I A and B molecules. Where there is a mismatch for KIRs between the donor and patient, the NK cells can kill residual leukaemia in the patient – a GvL effect. Laboratory tests have demonstrated that all CML and AML cells could be killed by alloreactive NK cells, whereas in ALL cells only a minority were killed. In autologous HSC transplants, NK cell activity can be stimulated by IL-2 treatment.

Table 19.5 Generation of cytotoxic T lymphocytes with leukaemia specificity.

Principle	Method	Specificity
Incubate DCs with apoptotic blast cells – blast cell lysates	Culture with autologous/ allogeneic lymphocytes	Unknown
Fuse normal DCs with blast cells	Culture with autologous/ allogeneic lymphocytes Inject directly to patient	Unknown
Culture blast cells with cytokine to produce 'leukaemic DCs'	Culture with autologous/ allogeneic lymphocytes Inject directly to patient	Unknown
Utilize the overexpression of antigens by leukaemic cells, e.g. Wilms' tumour 1 (WT-1)	Transfect TcR with WT-1 specificity into autologous T cells and inject these to patient	WT-1
Allotransplant: patient positive for a minor histocompatibility antigen, e.g. HA-1; donor is negative	Stimulate donor T cells to expand those recognizing HA-1 and infuse to patient	HA-1

DC, dendritic cell; TcR, T cell receptor.

T regulatory cells

These cells develop in the thymus and are essential for peripheral tolerance to self. They express CD4, CD25 (an activation marker) and a protein called Foxp3, and work via cell–cell contact. They may allow for activation of alloreactive T cells and therefore GvL responses, but prevent the massive expansion of T cells that causes GvHD. In keeping with this, patients with higher levels of T regulatory cells after HSC transplant were less likely to have GvHD.

Clinical protocols using immunotherapy

Leukaemia

A number of methods are being developed to generate CTLs with antileukaemia activity (Table 19.5).

Haemopoietic stem cell transplantation

Areas for possible immunotherapeutic intervention include:

1 Donor leucocyte infusions are used in the case of relapse in patients with CML, acute leukaemia and multiple myeloma.
2 Some transplant groups have shown that if CD8-positive T cells are depleted from *donor* leucocytes prior to infusion, then the GvL effect is preserved but less GvHD occurs.
3 Virus-specific CTLs can be infused to patients with post-transplant infections, e.g. CMV.
4 T regulatory cells can be used to modulate GvHD.

Solid tumours

Patients with renal, liver and prostate cancer and malignant melanoma are currently being given dendritic cells pulsed with tumour antigens and the regression of their disease studied.

Stem cell plasticity and non-haemopoietic stem cells

The potential of adult HSCs to regenerate all blood cells has been known for many decades and has been successfully applied to cure a variety of haematological disorders. Moreover, the plasticity of mammalian stem cells remains an area of controversy and intensive investigation.

There are two definitions of stem cell plasticity:

1 Stem cells are plastic in their ability to balance their self-renewal as undifferentiated cells with their capacity to differentiate into specific lineages.
2 The second concept is their ability to switch to lineages that they are not normally programmed to generate.

We can understand these concepts more easily if we apply them to two classes of stem cells: embryonic stem cells and 'tissue-specific' stem cells.

Embryonic stem cells can be derived from the inner cell mass of the blastocyst after fertilization and before implantation. These cells possess extensive self-renewal capacity and are able to give rise to identical offspring for many generations. They also have the potential to differentiate into mature cells. The most commonly used embryonic stem cell lines are those that have the potential to differentiate into the three germ layers – endoderm, mesoderm and ectoderm – and thus to generate most tissues in an organism. These cells may be regarded as truly 'plastic' as they not only have an enormous potential to regenerate undifferentiated stem cells, but are also able to switch into multiple somatic cell types found in the adult organism. Currently they are not used for clinical transplantation because of the need to further understand their differentiation potential *in vitro* and their functionality both *in vitro* and in pre-clinical trials, and to ensure their safety *in vivo* (i.e. that they do not form teratomas and that they mediate appropriate functional repair of tissues after transplantation).

Tissue-specific or 'adult' stem cells may be multipotent, but they have a much more restricted potential. Of those, HSCs still remain the best characterized adult mammalian stem cell type. Their major properties are:

- rarity (frequency <1 in 10^4 to 10^5 cells in tissues or blood)
- extensive proliferative capacity or ability to 'self-renew'
- ability to balance self-renewal with differentiation, ensuring a sustained stem cell population
- multipotency, i.e. a single HSC can give rise to 10–11 functional committed haemopoietic or blood cell lineages.

Newer concepts of stem cell plasticity imply the capability of stem cells to switch lineages and acquire the phenotype of a stem cell from a different tissue or organ from whence it is derived.

Bone marrow, fetal or cord blood derived HSCs have been reported to undergo a variety of conversions, where they differentiate into neural, cardiac muscle, liver, epithelial and skin cells, and even oocytes. An alternative explanation is that bone marrow, fetal blood or cord blood contains, in addition to HSCs, diverse stem cell types that mediate the effects described. These include: haemangioblasts or precursors for HSCs and endothelial stem cells, mesenchymal stem cells that are precursors for bone, cartilage, fat and haemopoietic and vascular supporting cells, and rare cells that resemble embryonic stem cells in their potentiality.

Besides haematological disorders, there is a group of human diseases for which stem cell-based therapies are likely to be beneficial in the future, such as Parkinson's disease, diabetes, bone and joint disorders, multiple sclerosis, cardiovascular diseases, cancer, etc. Therapies for bone, joint or heart disorders using cells from haemopoietic tissues are either in existence or are under development. The key challenges that we face relate to a detailed understanding of the diversity of the stem cells themselves. To be therapeutically useful, we need to know their concentration, function and potential in a particular tissue or cell line, their molecular signature or identity, their potential to develop abnormalities, their ease of collection, isolation, manipulation, expansion, differentiation and reprogramming, and *in vivo* function.

Conclusion

Expansion of the donor base, a wide use of mobilized peripheral blood cells and cord blood, and non-myeloablative conditioning transplantation marked a decade of important progress in haemopoietic cell transplantation, rendering it safer and available to more patients. There has been a paradigm shift from myeloablation of host cells to manipulation of immune mechanisms to support engraftment, exploit the antitumour potential of the graft, and provide cells capable of combating infectious agents. With more profound knowledge of stem cell biology, it might be possible to use stem cells derived from the bone marrow or blood for tissue repair in diverse conditions in the near future.

Further reading

Ballen KK. New trends in umbilical cord transplantation. *Blood* 2005; **105**: 3786–92. www.embt.org

Department of Health Code of Practice for Tissue Banks, www.dh.gov.uk

European Group for Blood and Marrow Transplantation, www.ebmt.org

Ljungman P et al. Allogeneic and autologous transplantation for haematological diseases, solid tumours and immune disorders: definitions and current practice in Europe. *Bone Marrow Transplantation* 2006; **37**: 439–49.

Burt RK, Loy Y, Pearce W et al. Clinical applications of blood-derived and marrow-derived stem cells for nonmalignant diseases. *Journal of the American Medical Association* 2008; **299**: 925–36.

CHAPTER 20

Blood Transfusion in a Regulatory Environment and the EU Directives

Shubha Allard, Clare Taylor and Angela Robinson

OVERVIEW

- Transfusion medicine is increasingly practised within a robust regulatory framework.

- The EU Directive on Blood Safety was written into UK Law as the Blood Safety and Quality Regulations 2005 with the Medicines and Healthcare Products Regulatory Agency as the competent authority.

- These regulations set standards of quality and safety for the collection, testing, processing, storage and distribution of blood and blood components.

- The key areas of impact for hospital transfusion laboratories include the need for a quality system, education and training, traceability of all blood and components transfused, and adverse event reporting via the SABRE online system.

- Only blood centres or hospital transfusion laboratories with blood establishment status can carry out processing of blood or components including irradiation.

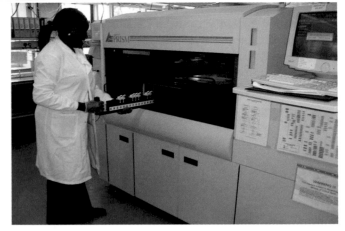

Figure 20.1 Automated microbiological testing. All donors are tested for hepatitis B and C, HIV, human T cell lymphotropic virus 1 and syphilis. Automation allows a rapid turnaround time for results. All techniques must be validated with clear documentation for compliance with the Blood Safety and Quality Regulations 2005.

Transfusion medicine in the UK and most developed countries is increasingly practised within a robust regulatory framework within a background of significant interest in the safety of blood and blood components with particular reference to transfusion-transmitted infection. The care delivered by the UK blood services and hospital transfusion laboratories to patients and donors is subjected to rigorous control within licensing and accreditation systems and within the principles of clinical governance. There is considerable emphasis on a code of good clinical practice including guidelines, quality systems, standard operating procedures, audit, good manufacturing practice and haemovigilance.

Why is regulation needed?

Both the practice of transfusion medicine and its service infrastructure have evolved rapidly over a few decades in line with scientific and clinical advances in the field. In order to achieve acceptable quality and safety for both donors and recipients of blood and

blood components, minimum standards of practice are needed. This is done by both internal audit and quality control as well as by external quality assessment, accreditation and inspection. External agencies involved in this process need to be empowered to enforce change in blood establishments or hospital laboratories that are found to be substandard.

Microbiological safety, especially related to hepatitis C, human immunodeficiency virus (HIV) (Figure 20.1) and new variant Creutzfeldt–Jakob disease (vCJD), has raised issues of national and international concern. More stringent donor selection criteria, new generations of serological tests with introduction of genomic testing, leucodepletion, viral inactivation processes, and testing for new pathogens have all been introduced. This in turn has fuelled debate in the transfusion world, the media and the law courts about the moral, medical and financial desirability of these interventions. Despite high court rulings in France and the UK a supply of 'risk free' blood components cannot, of course, be achieved. However standardization and regulation of the entire process – collection, testing, processing, storage and distribution – reduce the likelihood of donors or patients coming to harm, and ultimately provide the framework for 'standard current practice' in any future debate or litigation relating to new pathogens or newly available tests.

ABC of Transfusion, 4th edition, 2009. Edited by Marcela Contreras. © 2009 Blackwell Publishing, ISBN: 978-1-4051-5646-2.

Table 20.1 Legislation within the blood transfusion regulatory framework in the UK.

Act/Directive	Date	Summary of terms	Regulatory/monitoring body
Medicines Act	1968	Manufacturer's special licence needed for the collection, processing and issue of blood/blood products subject to inspection and demonstration of compliance with standards of good manufacturing practice. Failure to comply with regulations can result in closure of the organization with possible claims of negligence	Medicines and Healthcare Products Regulatory Agency (MHRA)
Consumer Protection Act	1987	Manufacturers (National Blood Service) and suppliers (hospital transfusion laboratories) are now considered liable if defective blood or blood product causes harm with no need to prove that any negligence took place. This has been the case since the successful litigation by patients infected with hepatitis C in 2001, where it was judged that blood should be regarded as a product and therefore subject to product liability under the Consumer Protection Act	
NHS Act Healthcare	1999	Places a statutory duty of quality on all NHS organizations promoting minimum standards of healthcare throughout the UK	Commission for Audit and Inspection (CHAI), also known as Healthcare Commission
European Union Blood Directive	2005	Transposed into UK law as the Blood Quality and Safety Regulations. All blood establishments must be regularly inspected and licensed by the MHRA. The National Blood Service and hospital transfusion laboratories must be registered and have demonstrated compliance against standards for collection, processing, storage and distribution of blood and blood products by return of a completed questionnaire with an inspection visit of some sites	MHRA

Table 20.2 Areas of impact of the EU regulations in the UK.

Processing – activities only allowed to take place in a BE, so work shifted from BB, with logistical, financial, staffing and training consequences	Washing cells, altering haematocrit, pooling of cryoprecipitate, granulocyte collection, preoperative autologous deposit, irradiation of components
Traceability – fully 'vein to vein' (donor to patient) in both directions, with records kept for 30 years (Figures 20.2–20.4)	System mostly in place for donors and BEs but documentation systems required in hospitals to document positively 'final fate' of components
Quality management systems	Requirement for full documentation at every stage, in line with the CPA and GMP standards 'Orange Book' and 'Red Book' (Figure 20.5). Records necessary in storage, cold chain, calibration and servicing of equipment in BBs
Adverse event reporting (Figure 20. 6)	Requirement for AE reports to go to CA first (not via SHOT) has resulted in a new SABRE system, which collates data required for EU commission as well as allowing full SHOT reporting
Training and education	Donor attendants, laboratory staff, clinical staff – porters, phlebotomists, nurses, doctors Documentation of all training

AE, adverse event; BB, blood bank; BE, blood establishment; CA, competent authority; CPA, clinical pathology accreditation; EU, European Union; GMP, good manufacturing practice; SABRE, Serious Adverse Blood Reactions and Events; SHOT, Serious Hazards of Transfusion.

Regulatory framework

The World Health Organization (WHO) and the Council of Europe (CoE) have recommended a code of ethical principles and guidelines for blood donation and transfusion practice and, while not legally binding, these formed the basis from which the standards were drafted for the subsequent European Union (EU) Directive on Blood Safety.

The various acts within the regulatory framework for blood transfusion are summarized in Table 20.1. The most recent of these, namely the EU Blood Directive, sets out far reaching and

legally binding regulations for the UK blood services and hospital transfusion laboratories (Table 20.2).

EU Blood Directive and the Blood Safety and Quality Regulations

The EU Directive on Blood Safety (2002/98/EC) set standards of quality and safety for the collection, testing, processing, storage and distribution of human blood and blood components. This was written into English law as the UK Blood Safety and Quality Regulations 2005, and was implemented in November 2005. In the UK, the 'competent authority' overseeing the implementation

STOP, SEE BACK OF THIS TAG BEFORE TRANSFUSION		**Compatibility and Traceability Tag**

STOP, SEE BACK OF THIS TAG BEFORE TRANSFUSION
Peel off label below and place in patients medical records
Donation number:
Component
Signature 1:
Signature 2: Date Given:
UNIT 1 of 4 Time Commenced
Surname: Forename:
Medical record number:
D.O.B: Gender
Patient Blood Group:

Once transfusion has finished you must complete the section below and return the whole tag to the Blood Transfusion Laboratory

This is a legal requirement

Surname:	Fore name:
Medical record number: (BARCODE)	
Donation number (BAR CODE)	
Component	Blood Group:
Date given:	Time completed:
I confirm that the above patient received this blood component Sign and print name	

Compatibility and Traceability Tag
PRE ADMINISTRATION

special requirements e.g. irradiate. Check concommitant drugs e.g diuretic

STEP 2: Check and document baseline observations

STEP 3: Check expiry date and time of component. Check pack for leaks, discolouration or clumping

ADMINISTRATION

STEP 1: Ask the patient their surname, forename and date of bith. Refer to hospital policy for unconscious or compromised patients

STEP 2: Check Surname, Forename, Date of Birth and patient identification number (MRN) against compatibility and traceability tag, patient notes and drug chart

STEP 3: Check that the information on the compatibility and traceability tag matches all the details on the blood component.

If there are any discrepancies <u>DO NOT PROCEED.</u>
Contact the Blood Transfusion Laboratory.

If you suspect a transfusion reaction – stop the transfusion immediately, contact medical staff, re check observations and compatibility

POST ADMINISTRATION

STEP 1: Detach purple self adhesive label (top of tag) and stick in patient notes

STEP 2: Complete date given the time completed sections in blue label (bottom), Sign and print name

STEP 3: Place whole tag in the specimen collection box

Under the Blood and safety quality regulations 2005

<u>IT IS A LEGAL REQUIREMENT</u>
that this section of the label must be completed and returned to the transfusion laboratory

Figure 20.2 Traceability tag. Paper systems for traceability of blood involve the use of a 'luggage label' attached to each unit. The details of the patient who receives the unit must be completed on the label by clinical staff and returned to the blood transfusion laboratory. The MHRA expects 100% compliance with traceability of blood and blood components.

of these regulations is currently the Medicines and Healthcare Products Regulatory Agency (MHRA; www.MHRA.gov.uk).

Implications of the new regulations for hospitals

The UK Blood Safety and Quality Regulations 2005 represent a significant change from past practices for hospitals, not least in the need for the chief executive to make a formal annual statement of compliance to the MHRA. The MHRA inspects and licences blood establishments regularly but can inspect hospital transfusion laboratories on an *ad hoc* basis if indicated and is empowered to give an order to 'cease and desist' (from) activities.

The UK Operational Impact Group (OIG) has advised hospitals on implementation of these regulations based on an assessment of current practice with priorities for action, together with potential resource implications including information technology (IT). The key areas of impact for hospitals are discussed below.

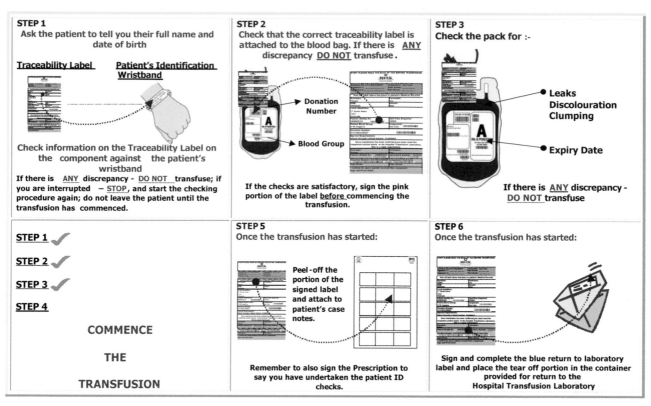

Figure 20.3 Traceability instructions. All clinical staff involved in blood transfusion must have training in maintaining traceability of all blood and blood components and this can be reinforced by use of training posters available in clinical areas. (Reproduced courtesy of the Scottish National Blood Service.)

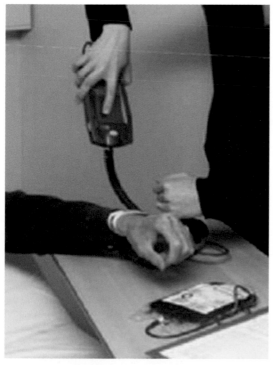

Figure 20.4 Electronic blood-tracking systems assist with the traceability of blood and can also be used for the electronic issue of blood at sites remote from the blood bank.

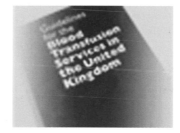

Figure 20.5 The 'Red Book' contains guidelines for all materials produced by the UK blood transfusion services for both therapeutic and diagnostic use. The guidelines reflect the legally binding requirements of the Blood Safety and Quality and Regulations 2005 (see www.transfusionguidelines.org.uk).

Quality systems

Hospital transfusion laboratories must have a comprehensive quality system in place based on the principles of 'good practice'. This includes stringent requirements for storage and distribution of blood and blood components with particular emphasis on 'cold chain' management together with validation and calibration of processes and equipment and change control. A designated quality manager is pivotal to the effective operation of a quality management system.

Traceability

The regulations require that hospitals must have complete traceability of the fate of each unit of blood/blood components (red

(a)

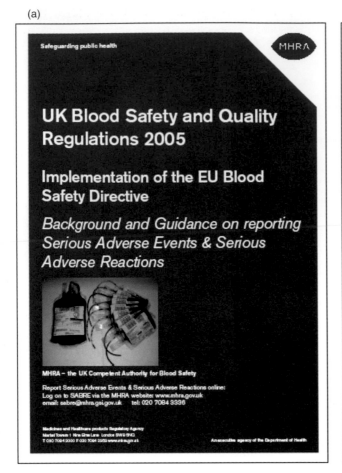

(b)

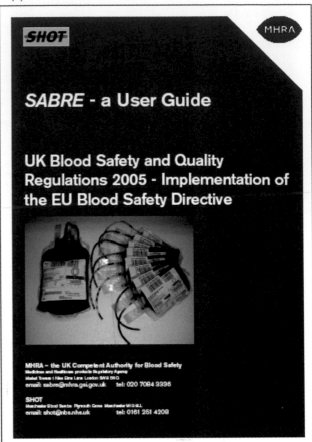

Figure 20.6 The UK Blood and Quality Safety Regulations 2005 require that serious adverse events and reactions related to transfusion of blood and blood components are reported to the MHRA. There are two guidance documents, namely (a) *Background and Guidance on reporting Serious Adverse Events and Serious Adverse Reactions* and (b) *SABRE – A User Guide* (see www.mhra.gov.uk).

cells, platelets, plasma and cryoprecipitate). These records must be kept for 30 years. The data set that is required for compliance includes: donation number, component type, identification of supplying blood establishment, transfused recipient identification, if not transfused, confirmation of final disposition, date of transfusion or final fate of component if not transfused.

Positive affirmation is required from all clinical areas regarding the fate of each unit of blood or blood component. The traceability information can be stored in a paper or electronic format but compliance must be 100%. Options for traceability systems include: (i) a paper-based system involving returning the label or signed paper document to the laboratory (Figures 20.2 and 20.3) and manual or electronic update of laboratory records; or (ii) a fully electronic system with barcode readers used by nursing and medical personnel when blood components are administered to patients (Figure 20.4). This would involve barcoded wrist identity bands for patients and additional hardware and software.

The OIG has stated that ultimately only effective electronic systems can ensure total traceability and recommends the inclusion of electronic blood tracking systems in the national IT programmes (e.g. Connecting for Health).

Education and training

All staff involved in the blood transfusion process must receive training and all training records must be available for inspection by the MHRA.

Haemovigilance

Adverse incidents must be reported as soon as known via the SABRE (Serious Adverse Blood Reactions and Events) online system hosted by the MHRA (Figure 20.6). This also includes online reporting to SHOT (Serious Hazards of Transfusion). See Chapter 15 for further details on haemovigilance.

Processing activities

The only processing activity that may be performed legally under these regulations by a hospital transfusion laboratory, is thawing of components (i.e. fresh frozen plasma and cryoprecipitate). Processing activities formerly undertaken in hospital transfusion laboratories but which are now permitted only in licensed blood establishments include irradiation, preoperative autologous deposit, granulocyte collection, splitting or pooling of components, and adjusting of haematocrit. Stem cell and donor lymphocyte collection, and intra- and postoperative cell salvage techniques, are excluded from the blood regulations, though stem cell and donor lymphocyte collection will be regulated under tissues legislation.

Amendments

Amendments based on Commission Directives 2005/61/EC and 2005/62/EC, containing further technical requirements with regard to blood and blood components, have been transposed into English law coming into force in August 2006. These have introduced further definitions for community facilities where blood may be transfused. The amendments also impose the requirement for hospital transfusion laboratories to have a system of traceability and to comply with the quality system requirements of Commission Directive 2005/62/EC. Transfusion laboratories are required to retain records of any serious adverse events that may affect the quality or safety of blood and blood components for at least 15 years.

Implications of the new regulations for blood establishments

Unlike hospital transfusion laboratories, blood establishments were already regulated by the MHRA and undergoing regular inspections. The secretary of state, via its 'competent authority', can grant a blood establishment licence to existing hospital transfusion laboratories to carry out processing activities (e.g. irradiation or granulocyte collection) with the newly licensed facility being inspected every 2 years.

The regulations set out details of the quality system and traceability requirements for blood establishments as well as requirements for testing and specifications for blood components and their labelling. An annual report must be sent to the EU via the competent authority with details of testing, including additional testing for epidemiological reasons, compliance with the quality system, including storage, transport and distribution conditions, and donor information and recruitment details.

Other standards and guidelines

There are several other sources of regulations and guidelines encompassing standards for the practice of clinical blood transfusion.

Better Blood Transfusion

Although not part of the regulatory framework, the two Health Service circulars, published in 1998 and 2002, with further update in 2007, have helped to ensure that the Better Blood Transfusion initiative is an integral part of NHS practice with responsibility firmly in the hands of NHS Trust management as part of the clinical governance structure. The key objectives include avoidance of unnecessary transfusion and making transfusion practice safer with better information for patients and the public. These initiatives have been discussed in detail in Chapter 19.

NHS Litigation Authority

The NHS Litigation Authority (NHSLA) is a Special Health Authority, responsible for handling negligence claims made against NHS bodies in England. Although membership of the scheme is voluntary, the majority of NHS Trusts (including

Foundation Trusts) currently belong to the scheme. Discounts are available to those trusts that achieve the relevant NHSLA risk management standards and these include blood transfusion practice.

Clinical Pathology Accreditation scheme

The Clinical Pathology Accreditation (CPA) scheme, introduced to UK pathology laboratories in 1992, is an external audit of the ability to provide a service of high quality and is confirmed by peer review. There are objective standards for all aspects of hospital laboratory work including blood transfusion laboratories, such as staffing, procurement and maintenance of equipment, use of standard operating procedures, reporting of results, internal audit, and external quality assessment with emphasis on continual quality improvement.

National Patient Safety Agency Safer Practice Notice

The National Patient Safety Agency (NPSA) was established in 2001 as a Special Health Authority with the aim of making the NHS 'an organisation with a memory', which learns from its mistakes via reporting and analysis of adverse events and near miss incidents.

Although not a regulation, the NPSA Safer Practice Notice *Right Patient – right blood* (NPSA 2006) has important implications for hospitals. The emphasis is on the final pre-transfusion bedside check, the need to consider information technology to improve transfusion safety, and the need for training and regular competency testing for all relevant staff involved in the transfusion process (including phlebotomists, blood transfusion laboratory staff, porters, nurses and medical staff).

Where next with regulation?

The Treaty of Amsterdam in 2000 empowered the European Parliament to legislate on the quality and safety of organs and substances of human origin, blood and blood derivatives. The outcome to date has been the EU Directive on Blood Safety and the Tissues and Cells Directive.

In the field of blood safety there are two outstanding areas that the EU had originally planned future action in:
1 Educational programmes for health professionals in the optimal use of blood.
2 The promotion of public information/education on blood collection and transfusion.

There will be commission follow-up of the implementation of the EU Blood Directives in community states. Action is being taken to standardize the training of inspectors, with the potential aim of a European-wide inspection system for blood services.

It can be anticipated that sooner or later proposals will be drawn up for the regulation of organ donation. However, article 152 of the Treaty of Amsterdam places some restriction on what the EU can legislate. The relevant clause states: 'community action in the field of public health shall respect the responsibilities of Member States for the organisation and delivery of health services and medical care, in particular measures shall not affect national provisions on donations or medical use of organs and blood'. In other words, at present the EU cannot legislate on the delivery of clinical services.

Whilst harmonization and regulation of quality and safety standards for these 'substances of human origin' is to be welcomed, the UK concern is that where the technical details are overproscriptive they are likely to need regular and occasionally rapid updating to respond to advances in knowledge and technology. The EU regulatory committee procedures necessary to make amendments to any of the EU Blood Directives is yet to be tested. Should this regulatory committee review process take too long, there is the potential for an adverse impact on quality and safety of 'substances of human origin' with the law requiring compliance with outdated standards.

Further reading

Murphy M, Pamphilon DH. *Practical Transfusion Medicine*. Blackwell Publishing, Oxford, 2005.
Operational Impact Group. *OIG Report*. www.transfusionguidelines.org.uk, under new regulations.

References

Department of Health. *Better Blood Transfusion*. HSC 1998/224. Department of Health, London, 1998.
Department of Health. *Better Blood Transfusion: appropriate use of blood*. HSC 2002/009. Depa rtment of Health, London, 2002.
Department of Health. *Better Blood Transfusion: safe and appropriate use of blood*. HSC 2007/001. Department of Health, London, 2007.
European Parliament and Council. Implementing Directive 2002/98/EC as regards standards of quality and safety for the collection, testing, processing, storage and distribution of human blood and blood components. *Office Journal of the European Union* 2003; L33/30.
European Parliament and Council. Implementing Directive 2005/61/EC as regards traceability requirements and notification of serious adverse reactions and events. *Office Journal of the European Union* 2005; L256/32.
European Parliament and Council. Implementing Directive 2005/62/EC as regards community standards and specifications relating to a quality system for blood establishments. *Office Journal of the European Union* 2005; L256/41.
National Patient Safety Agency (NPSA). *Right Patient – right blood*. NPSA/2006/14. National Patient Safety Agency 2006, www.npsa.nhs.uk.
UK Blood Safety and Quality Regulations 2005. Statutory Instrument 2005, No. 50. © Crown Copyright 2005. www.opsi.gov.uk/si/si2005/20050050.htm.

Index

Note: Page numbers in **bold** represent tables, those in *italics* represent figures.

117